W9-BIB-418

Herbal Antibiotics

Natural Alternatives

for Treating

Drug-Resistant

Bacteria

Stephen Harrod Buhner

Foreword by James A. Duke, Ph.D.

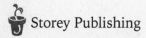 Storey Publishing

*The mission of Storey Publishing is to serve our customers
by publishing practical information that encourages
personal independence in harmony with the environment.*

Edited by Deborah Balmuth
Cover design by Meredith Maker
Cover art production and text design by Betty Kodela
Text production by Susan Bernier
Illustrations by Beverly Duncan, except on pages 1, 23, 33, 57, and 102 by Sarah Brill; pages 18, 49, 60, 87, and 93 by Brigita Fuhrmann; and pages 26, 89, and 91 by Alison Kolesar
Indexed by Peggy Holloway
Professional review by David Hoffmann

ISBN-13: 978-1-58017-148-9
Printed in the United States by R.R. Donnelley

DEDICATION

Rosemary Gladstar, Susun Weed, and David Hoffmann — for knowing (and living) that it is essential to risk exposing the deepest weaknesses of the self for the work that we are here to do to come through. Matthew Wood — for having the courage to begin finding a unique Western herbal diagnostic system and for being the first to publicly say that Samuel Thompson knew what he was doing. Mary Shelley — for bringing the dangers of our times so clearly into story form and into our collective consciousness.

ACKNOWLEDGMENTS

Thanks to Barbara Griggs for the Latin quotation in the Epilogue which is from the Middle Ages text, *A Treatise on Scurvy.* Thanks are also due to Paul Bergner and K. P. Khalsa for the excellence of their clinical work and research, and to Marc Lappé for understanding that bacterial resistance is an ecological and not an overuse problem.

CONTENTS

Foreword by James A. Duke, Ph.D. v

Preface vii

1 The End of Antibiotics? 1

2 Botanical Medicines with the
  Strongest Antibiotic Properties 18

3 The First Line of Defense:
  Strengthening the Immune System 67

4 Making and Using Herbal Medicines 85

Epilogue 106

Glossary 107

Resources 110

Suggested Reading 110

Selected Bibliography 110

General References 127

Index 128

FOREWORD

by James A. Duke, Ph.D.

Stephen Buhner has arrived at (and shares with you, the reader) the frightening truth that you won't find in the *Journal of the American Medical Association:* We are running out of weapons in the war on germs. Since germs can go through a generation in 20 minutes or so, instead of the 20 years or so it takes us humans to reproduce ourselves, it's no small wonder that the germs are evolving resistance to our chemical weapons as rapidly as we develop them.

When the drug vancomycin falls completely by the wayside, as it will, we may, just as Stephen predicts here and I have predicted elsewhere, fall back on the bimillennial biblical medicinal herbs such as garlic and onion. These herbs each contain dozens of mild antibiotic compounds (some people object to using the term "antibiotic" to refer to higher plant phytochemicals, but I do not share their disdain for such terminology). It is easy for a rapidly reproducing bug or bacterial species to outwit (out-evolve) a single compound by learning to break it down or even to use it in its own metabolism, but not so easy for it to outwit the complex compounds found in herbs. Scientists are recognizing this fact and developing more complex compounds such as the AIDS cocktail and multiple chemotherapies for cancer. The same super-scientists who downplay the herbalists' claims of synergies that account for the effectiveness of particular herbs and herbal formulas, are now resorting to synergies of three or four compounds in their pharmaceutical formulas.

It is certainly easier to demonstrate how two compounds can work synergistically than it is to figure out how 200 or 2000 different compounds (and more, as are present in all herbs) can work synergistically.

So, the scientific community will be reluctant to consider the remarkable synergistic suites of compounds that have evolved naturally in plants. But we really cannot afford to ignore these. For nature favors synergies among beneficial, plant-protective compounds within a plant species (with antibacterial, antifeedant, antifungal, antiviral, and insecticidal properties), and selects against antagonisms.

When we borrow the antibiotic compounds from plants, we do better to borrow them all, not just the single solitary most powerful among them. We lose the synergy when we take out the solitary compound. But most important we facilitate the enemy, the germ, in its ability to outwit the monochemical medicine. The polychemical synergistic mix, concentrating the powers already evolved in medicinal plants, may be our best hope for confronting drug-resistant bacteria.

THE EVOLUTION OF "MODERN" MEDICINE
(as imagined and adapted by Jim Duke from Internet surf castings)

8,000,000 years ago: One chimp to another: "I have a tummy ache . . ." *(in chimpanzeze, rubbing tummy).* Response: "Here, chimp, eat these bitter herbs!" *(in chimpanzeze)*

5,000,000 years ago: "Here, Hominid, eat these bitter herbs" *(in hominidese)*

2,500,000 years ago: "Here, Homo, eat these bitter herbs and leave some for the Leakeys to find!" *(in humanoid sign language)*

2500 B.C.: "Here man, eat these bitter herbs!" *(in Arabic, Coptic, Farsi, Hebrew, etc.).*

A.D. 0: "The saviour is borne! Faith can heal. Eat these bitter herbs (if faith should fail!)."

A.D. 1200: "Those bitter herbs aren't Christian. Say a prayer when you take those bitters!"

A.D. 1850: "That prayer is superstition. Here, drink this bitter potion!"

A.D. 1900: "That bitter potion is snake oil. Here, swallow this bitter pill!"

A.D. 1950: "That bitter pill is ineffective. Here, take this bitter antibiotic!"

A.D. 2000: "That bitter antibiotic is artificial, ineffective, and toxic; besides all the microbes are resistant, and some even feed on it (even vancomycin). Here, eat these bitter herbs. And pray they will help you (95 percent of Americans, but only 33 percent of psychologists, are reported to pray)."

PREFACE

I came to herbal medicine as many of us do: I became ill, and modern medicine could not help me. I felt betrayed. I was shocked, then angry. Then I began to think about a great many things in new ways.

Because I was raised in a family of powerful political physicians, I was raised with the belief that after millennia, man (and modern medical science) had defeated disease. I was taught to believe that we were all on the threshold of everlasting, disease-free life. It was a tremendous shock, then, when reality took me aside and whispered in my ear. That murmured secret was an antibiotic-resistant ear infection. My physician at the time leafed futilely through pharmaceutical advertising circulars, trying one antibiotic after another to no avail. Unknown to both of us, all that we were doing was killing off the friendly bacteria in my body and leaving the way open to the antibiotic-resistant strain to multiply unhindered.

Eventually I turned to herbs for treatment when it was clear that pharmaceuticals could not help. And, as they often do, herbal medicines worked. This was not the first time the plant world had cured what, for me, was a painful disease. But it was the final catalyst that caused me to abandon modern approaches and enter fully into the plant world. It was also the catalyst for my interest in epidemic disease and antibiotic-resistant bacteria.

In the many years since that painful event, I have continued to deepen my knowledge and interest in such bacteria, and to write and speak often about them. They fascinate me. They are also the origin of a deepening humility. The two great lessons they have taught me are that human arrogance about the natural world has an inevitable, unpleasant outcome and that this sacred Earth upon which we live, without fanfare or personal aggrandizement, offers to humankind medicines with which to treat the bacterial superbugs that we, in our arrogance, have created. Like so many people before me, I had always known that I should work to save the Earth. I never knew before my illness that it was a two-way street: that the Earth also works to save us.

This book explores some of the realities of antibiotic-resistant bacteria and some of the most powerful herbal medicines with which to treat them. In the coming years, I think many of us will need to understand both. I hope that for you, as it has been for me, this knowledge will be useful.

1

THE END OF ANTIBIOTICS?

There is a unique smell to hospitals, composed of equal parts illness, rubbing alcohol, fear, and hope. Few of us who have been in a hospital can forget that smell or the feelings it engenders. But underneath those memory-laden smells and feelings is the belief that in this place, this hospital, there is an army of men and women fighting for our lives, working to bring us back from the brink of death. We have learned, been taught, know, that this army is winning the war against disease, that antibiotics have made an end to most bacterial diseases. It is a comforting belief. Unfortunately, what we "know" couldn't be more wrong.

Late in 1993, as *Newsweek*'s Sharon Begley reported, infectious disease specialist Dr. Cynthia Gilbert entered the room of a patient with a long-term kidney condition. Her face was set in the mask that physicians have used for centuries when coming to pass sentence on their patients. The man was not fooled; he took it in at a glance.

"You're coming to tell me I'm dying," he said.

She paused, then nodded curtly. "There's just nothing we can do."

They each paused, then. One contemplating the end of life; the other, the failure of her craft and the loss that goes with it.

Dr. Gilbert took a deep and shuddering breath. "I'm sorry," she said.

The man said nothing; for what he was contemplating, there were no words. His physician nodded sharply as if settling her mind. Then she turned and left him, facing once again the long hall filled with the smells of illness, rubbing alcohol, fear, hope, and questions for which she had no answer.

Her patient was going to die of something easily curable a few years earlier — an enterococcus bacterial infection. But this particular bacterium was now resistant to antibiotics; for nine months she had tried every antibiotic in her arsenal. The man, weakened as he was by disease, could not fight off bacteria that were impervious to pharmaceuticals. Several days later, he succumbed to a massive infection of the blood and heart.

This picture, inconceivable a decade ago, is growing ever more common. Some three million people a year are admitted to hospitals with difficult-to-treat resistant infections, and another two million (5 percent of hospital patients) become infected while visiting hospitals for routine medical procedures. More and more of these patients are succumbing to disease as the virulence and resistance of bacteria increase. In fact, as pathologist and author Marc Lappé of the University of Illinois College of Medicine observes, "by conservative estimate, such infections are responsible for at least a hundred thousand deaths a year, and the toll is mounting." The toll is mounting because the number of people infected by resistant bacteria is increasing, especially in places where the ill, the young or old, or the poor congregate, such as homeless shelters, hospitals, inner cities, prisons, and child care centers. Perhaps the best-known and most-loved casualty to date is Jim Henson, the creator of Kermit the Frog, who died in 1990. In the face of the enormous inroads that resistant bacteria are making, world-renowned authority on bacterial resistance, Dr. Stuart Levy, comments, "This situation raises the staggering possibility that a time will come when antibiotics as a mode of therapy will be only a fact of historic interest." Marc Lappé is more blunt: "The period once euphemistically called the Age of Miracle Drugs is dead." Humankind now faces the threat of epidemic diseases more powerful, and less treatable, than any known before.

> We have let our profligate use of antibiotics reshape the evolution of the microbial world and wrest any hope of safe management from us. . . . Resistance to antibiotics has spread to so many different, and such unanticipated types of bacteria, that the only fair appraisal is that we have succeeded in upsetting the balance of nature.
>
> MARC LAPPÉ, PH.D., AUTHOR OF
> WHEN ANTIBIOTICS FAIL

Many people are now asking themselves how this could have happened; only a few short years ago, the picture seemed decidedly different.

In the late 1950s and early 1960s, my great-uncle Leroy Burney, then Surgeon General of the United States, and my grandfather David Cox, president of the Kentucky Medical Association, joined many other physicians in the industrialized nations in declaring that the antibiotic era had come, jointly proclaiming the end for all time of epidemic disease.

This 1962 statement by an eminent Nobel laureate, the Australian physician Sir F. Macfarlane Burnet, is typical. By the end of the twentieth century, he commented, we will see the "virtual elimination of infectious disease as a significant factor in societal life." Further study and publication of infectious disease research, he continued, "is almost to write of something that has passed into history." Seven years later, one of my great-uncle's successors, Surgeon General William Stewart, testified to Congress that "it was time to close the book on infectious diseases." They couldn't have been more wrong.

THE END OF MIRACLE DRUGS

Though penicillin was discovered in 1928, only during World War II was it commercially developed, and not until after the war did its use became routine. Those were heady days. It seemed that science could do anything. New antibiotics were being discovered daily; the arsenal of medicine seemed overwhelming. In the euphoria of the moment, no one heeded the few voices raising concerns. Among them, ironically enough, was Alexander Fleming, the discoverer of penicillin. Dr. Fleming noted as early as 1929 in the *British Journal of Experimental Pathology* that numerous bacteria were already resistant to the drug he had discovered, and by 1945 he warned in a *New York Times* interview that improper use of penicillin would inevitably lead to the development of resistant bacteria. Fleming's observations were only too true. At the time of his interview, just 14 percent of *Staphylococcus aureus* bacteria were resistant to penicillin. By 1950, an incredible 59 percent were resistant, and by 1995, that figure had jumped to 95 percent. Originally limited to patients in the hospitals (the primary breeding ground for such bacteria), the resistant strains are now common throughout the world's population. And though many factors influence the growth of resistant bacteria, the most important are ecological.

Throughout our history on this planet, our species has lived in an ecological balance with many other life-forms, including the bacterial. Epidemic diseases did flash through the human population from time to time, usually in response to local overpopulation or unsanitary conditions. But epidemics like the bubonic plague that decimated Europe were relatively uncommon. At the end of World War II, this relationship was significantly altered when antibiotics were introduced. For the first time in human history, the microbial world was intentionally being affected on a large scale. In the heady euphoria of discovery, an ancient human hubris again raised its head when science declared war on bacteria. And like all wars, this one is likely to cause the deaths of thousands, if not millions, of noncombatants.

> Such vehement antipathy toward any corner of the living world should have given us pause. Through our related mistakes in the world of higher animals, we should have gained the evolutionary wisdom to predict the outcome.
>
> *MARC LAPPÉ, PH.D.*

Evolution of Antibiotic Use

Though it is not commonly known, our ancestors had used both penicillin and tetracycline in raw form, as bread mold or as soil fungi, directly on wounds or even ingested to treat disease. As physician Stuart Levy reveals in his book *The Antibiotic Paradox,* thousand-year-old Nubian mummies have been found to have significant amounts of tetracycline in their systems. Even though several of the antibiotics we now use come from such naturally occurring organisms, they are usually refined into a single substance, a silver bullet, a form not normally present in nature. And the quantities being produced are staggering.

In December 1942, almost the entire manufactured supply of penicillin — 8½ gallons (32 liters) — was used to treat the survivors of the Coconut Grove restaurant fire. By 1949, 156 thousand pounds (70,762 kg) a year of penicillin and a new antibiotic, streptomycin, were being produced. By 1992, *in the United States alone,* this figure grew to an incredible 40 million pounds (18,144,000 kg) a year of scores of antibiotics. Most of these newer antibiotics are synthesized and do not occur naturally. Stuart Levy comments that "these antibiotics can remain intact in the environment unless they are destroyed by high temperatures or other physical damage such as ultraviolet light from the sun. As active antibiotics they continue to kill off susceptible bacteria with which they have contact." To put it another way, we are putting increasingly large numbers of antibacterial substances into the environment without regard to the consequences. Few people understand the quantity of antibiotics being used each year, and even fewer have thought of the potential environmental (not just human) consequences. For instance, the soil fungi that produce tetracycline do so to protect themselves from aggressive bacteria. Those particular soil fungi play a significant part in the health of the Earth's soil. That many bacteria are now resistant to tetracycline has been viewed with alarm because of the potential impact on *our* health. But what about the health of that original soil fungus from which tetracycline came? How about the mold that makes penicillin to protect itself from aggressive bacteria? How about the many other members of the ecosystem that taught us to make many of the antibiotics we use? How are they faring? And how about the health of our entire ecosystem if the balance between bacteria and all other organisms becomes too one-sided?

Many scientists now realize that any attempt to destroy all disease organisms along with which we inhabit this planet was doomed to failure from the start. There is a *reason* for everything in the ecosystem. As Marc Lappé observes, in the race to destroy disease, "an absurd pharmaceutical morality play unfolded: we became soldiers against implacable microscopic enemies with which we actually co-evolved. Only recently have a few scientists pointed out that the survival of bacteria as a group underlies our own." We cannot pick and choose which bacteria we decide to war on and kill off. They are all an inextricable part of a healthy ecosystem. Lappé continues, "The lesson from both our agricultural and medical experience is remarkable for its consistency: Ignoring the evolutionary attributes of biological systems can only be done at the peril of ecological catastrophe." Stuart Levy agrees: "Antibiotic usage has stimulated evolutionary changes that are unparalleled in recorded biologic history." Bacteria, evolving at pretty much a constant pace along with the rest of us, are now changing at an ever faster rate, and they are changing in ways that scientists once insisted were impossible. They are, in fact, developing resistance to the incredible quantities of antibiotics we are pouring into the ecosystem, and they are doing so in ways that show they are highly intelligent and adaptable.

HOW BACTERIA DEVELOP RESISTANCE

When we are born we are sterile; there are *no* bacteria on or in our bodies. Normally the first thing that happens after birth is that we are placed on our mother's stomach and we begin to nurse. At this moment our skin begins to be colonized with human-friendly bacteria from our mother's body, and our intestinal tract begins to be colonized from bacteria from our mother's milk.

Eventually, 1 to 2 pounds (½ to 1 kg) of our mature body weight will be the billions of bacteria that live in healthy symbiosis in and on our bodies. Many of these bacteria produce essential nutrients that we could not live without. Even more striking, researchers are discovering that many of these friendly bacteria actually fight off more dangerous bacteria in order to keep us healthy. Babies removed from their mothers before this healthy colonization can take place (usually in hospitals) are often colonized with bacteria that are anything but friendly to human beings. Eventually, there are literally billions of bacteria on and in our bodies at any one time. Most of these bacteria are friendly to us; a few are not. These unfriendly or pathogenic bacteria usually remain in small numbers and, in general, do us no harm.

But when we become ill, the ecological balance in our body is disturbed, and some of the friendly bacteria are displaced enough to allow pathogenic bacteria to gain a toehold. As our body tries to throw off the infection we show classic symptoms of disease, such as fever, chills, vomiting, or diarrhea. In some cases we then go to a doctor and are given antibiotics to kill the disease organisms. However, there is not just one kind of that particular disease bacterium in our bodies; there are many, a few of which are naturally immune or resistant to antibiotics. Generally, these few resistant bacteria are in competition with their nonresistant cousins (and all the other helpful bacteria) for living space in

> Antibiotic usage has stimulated evolutionary changes that are unparalleled in recorded biologic history.
>
> *Stuart Levy, M.D.*

our bodies. But when antibiotics are used they kill off the nonresistant disease bacteria (and often many or most of the other, helpful bacteria), leaving the resistant bacteria to reproduce without competition. The resistant bacteria then take over our body without hindrance. As this process occurs with more and more people these resistant bacteria begin passing into the general human population. Eventually, most pathogenic bacteria end up immune to commonly used antibiotics. The susceptible ones have all been killed off.

In a way, we have created a kind of evolution in fast forward. We have supported a bacterial survival-of-the-fittest through our creation and use of pharmaceuticals. But the truth is even more complex, and frightening, than this picture reveals. For evolution, long thought to be merely a passive process — the fastest gazelle surviving to have babies, for instance — is much more complex indeed.

Adapting to Survive Antibiotics

What our forefathers failed to understand in those heady decades of the 1940s and 1950s is that bacteria are a life-form, and like all life they have the drive to survive and reproduce. And like all life they adapt to threats to their survival. Not only are some bacteria naturally immune to antibiotics, but all of them respond remarkably quickly to changes in their environment. They are pure biochemical factories that respond to antibiotics with metabolic changes in an attempt to counter them. In other words, bacteria use a kind of trial-and-error process to create chemical responses to antibiotics. These chemicals allow them to survive antibiotics or even to disable the antibiotic itself. As physician Jeffery Fisher observes:

> Bacteria don't do this instantly, but rather through evolutionary trial and error. Once the right biochemical combination to resist the antibiotic in question develops, the new mutated strain will flourish — a pure example of Darwinian survival of the fittest. Trial and error, of course, can take time, generally bacterial generations. Here again, however, the bacteria prove to have the perfect machinery. Unlike humans, who produce a new generation every twenty years or so, bacteria produce a new generation every twenty minutes, multiplying 500,000 times faster than we do.

And not only do the bacteria, those naturally immune and those mutating, survive the antibiotics, many also seem to get stronger so that the diseases they cause are more severe and generate greater mortality than those they produced before. We have been, in fact, creating what *The New York Times* is now calling bacterial superbugs. But as incredible as this capacity for literally engineering responses to antibiotics and passing it on to their offspring is, bacteria do something else that makes them even more amazing and dangerous. They communicate intelligently with each other. It has taken scientists a long time to discover this. We were raised to believe that bacteria are pretty dumb, but it is turning out that the other life-forms with which we share this planet are much smarter than we gave them credit for. And bacteria are turning out to be very smart indeed.

Communicating Resistance

Bacteria are single-cell organisms containing, among other things, special loops of their DNA called plasmids. Whenever two bacteria meet — and they do not have to be the same kind of bacteria — they position themselves alongside each other and exchange information. Bacteria, in fact, possess a kind of biological Internet, and these information exchanges occur with great frequency. Unfortunately for us, one of the types of information they exchange is antibiotic resistance.

During an information exchange, a resistant bacterium extrudes a filament of itself, a plasmid, to the nonresistant bacterium, which opens a door in its cell wall. Within the filament is a copy of a portion of the resistant bacterium's DNA. Specifically, it contains the encoded information on resistance to one or more antibiotics. This DNA copy is now a part of the new bacterium; it is now resistant to all the antibiotics the first bacterium was resistant to. It can pass this resistance on to its offspring or to any other bacteria it meets. This communicated resistance can be a natural immunity, information on how to disable or destroy a particular antibiotic or antibiotics, or information on how to prevent the antibiotic from having an effect. And bacteria that have never been known to communicate — gram-negative and gram-positive bacteria, aerobic and nonaerobic bacteria, for instance — have seemingly learned the art. Bacteria are in fact intelligently communicating to each other how best to fight the weapons we have created to destroy them. As Dr. Richard Wenzel of the University of Iowa commented in *Newsweek,* "They're so much older than we are . . . and wiser."

If this were the end of it, it would be bad enough, but our intervention into the microbial sphere has created even more responses from bacteria than we thought possible.

Bacteria that have the ability to resist antibiotics are now known to emit unique pheromones to attract bacteria to themselves in order to exchange resistant information. It is almost as if they put up a sign that says "bacterial resistance information here." More, the seminal discoveries of genetic researcher Barbara McClintock are also at work. Bacteria, like corn, also possess "jumping genes," or transposons, that are able to jump from bacterium to bacterium independently of plasmid exchange. These transposons also have the ability to "teach" antibiotic resistance. Furthermore, bacteria also have diseases: bacterial viruses (called bacteriophages). These viruses, as they infect other bacteria, pass on the information for resistance. Finally, bacteria release free-roving pieces of their DNA, which carry resistance information. Other bacteria that encounter it ingest it, thereby learning how to survive antibiotics. Yet, even with all this, there is still more that they do.

In ways no researcher understands, bacteria learn resistance to multiple antibiotics *from encountering only one antibiotic.* Medical researchers have placed bacteria into solutions containing *only* tetracycline in such a way that the bacteria are not killed; they live in a tetracycline-heavy environment. In short order the bacteria develop resistance to tetracycline, but they also develop resistance to other antibiotics that they have never encountered. And being isolated, they have never come into contact with resistance information from other bacteria. Levy comments that "it's almost as if bacteria strategically anticipate the confrontation of other drugs when they resist one."

This uncanny ability of bacteria to develop immunity, their ever more rapid manner of learning it, and the almost supernatural appearance of resistance in bacteria that haven't had exposure to specific antibiotics leads Levy to remark that "one begins to see bacteria, not as individual species, but as a vast array of interacting constituents of an integrated microbial world." Or, as former FDA commissioner Donald Kennedy remarked, "The evidence indicates that enteric microorganisms in animals and man, their R plasmids, and human pathogens form a linked ecosystem of their own in which action at any one point can affect every other." So wherever pathogenic bacteria encounter the regular use of antibiotics, they learn, and adapt, and become resistant.

Places of Transmission

The worst offenders of antibiotic overuse have been hospitals, and it is here that the majority of bacteria have learned resistance and entered the general population. Many of the bacteria have learned to be population specific. In hospitals, resistant bacteria such as enterococcus, *Pseudomonas, Staphylococcus,* and *Klebsiella* take advantage of surgical procedures to infect surgical wounds or the blood (bacteremia). Some, such as *Haemophilus, Pseudomonas, Staphylococcus, Klebsiella,* and *Streptococcus,* cause severe, often untreatable pneumonia (especially in elderly patients in hospitals or nursing homes). *Haemophilus* and *Streptococcus* also cause serious ear infections (usually in day care centers), sometimes leading to meningitis. *Pseudomonas* and *Klebsiella* also cause serious urinary tract infections (usually in hospital patients and female nurses, who then spread them to the general population). Tuberculosis, long thought conquered, is increasingly resistant and is occurring more and more frequently in places where large numbers of people are confined for long periods of time, such as prisons and homeless shelters, and in large cities. Gonorrhea has emerged as a potent resistant disease throughout the world, learning resistance in brothels in Vietnam among prostitutes who were regularly given antibiotics. Malaria, spread by mosquitoes and usually considered a disease of the tropics, learned resistance in crowded Asia and is making inroads in the United States in such unlikely places as Minnesota and New York. Malaria, in fact, is becoming so serious a problem in the United States that in August 1997, the *Atlantic Monthly* featured an article on the disease as its lead cover story. But still other resistant bacteria have entered the human disease picture from a different and nonhuman source: huge agribusiness factory farms.

12 MOST COMMON DRUG-RESISTANT BACTERIA

All bacteria will eventually learn resistance, and there are thousands if not millions of species. These are the most resistant or problematic of those that cause human disease.

BACTERIUM	DISEASES IT CAUSES
Enterococcus	Bacteremia, surgical and urinary tract infections
Haemophilus influenzae	Meningitis, ear infections, pneumonia, sinusitis, epiglottitis
Mycobacterium tuberculosis	Tuberculosis
Neisseria gonorrhoeae	Gonorrhea
Plasmodium falciparum	Malaria
Pseudomonas aeruginosa	Bacteremia, pneumonia, urinary tract infections
Shigella dysenteriae	Severe diarrhea
Staphylococcus aureus	Bacteremia, pneumonia, surgical wound infections
Streptococcus pneumoniae	Meningitis, pneumonia, ear infections
Klebsiella pneumoniae	Bacteremia, pneumonia, urinary tract and surgical wound infections
Escherichia coli	Severe or bloody diarrhea
Salmonella	Severe diarrhea

A note on classifying bacteria: Bacteria are classified as either gram-negative or gram-positive bacteria, so denoted because of the way their cell membranes take a stain (positive) or don't (negative). The gram-positive bacteria are enterococcus, *Mycobacterium tuberculosis, Staphylococcus aureus,* and *Streptococcus pneumoniae.* The gram-negative bacteria are *Shigella dysenteriae, Haemophilus influenzae, Neisseria gonorrhoeae,* and *Pseudomonas aeruginosa.*

THE GROWTH OF RESISTANT STRAINS IN FACTORY FARMS

Unknown to most of us, huge agribusinesses took advantage of early experiments that showed that farm animals regularly fed subclinical doses of antibiotics experienced faster growth. The pharmaceutical companies, too, were excited at this research. Not only could they sell increasing amounts of antibiotics for use as medicine, they could now branch out into the food supply for a fast-growing population. Thousands of tons — in fact, half of all the antibiotics used in the United States (some 20 million pounds [9,072,000 kg] a year) — are fed to farm animals as a routine part of their diet. The antibiotics force growth (something that overcrowding traditionally inhibits) and reduce disease (a common problem when any life-form is overcrowded). As always, bacteria began to learn, and they learned fast. Three of them threaten exceptionally serious human infections: *E. coli* O157:H7 in beef, *Salmonella* in chicken eggs, and *Campylobacter* in chickens. (And there are others, such as *Cyclospora, Cryptosporidium, Listeria,* and *Yersinia.*) According to Nicols Fox, in her exposé of the problem in her book *Spoiled: The Dangerous Truth about a Food Chain Gone Haywire:*

> The conditions under which [farm animals were] raised presented all the conditions for infection and disease: the animals were closely confined; subjected to stress; often fed contaminated food and water; exposed to vectors (flies, mice, rats) that could carry contaminants from one flock to another; bedded on filth-collecting litter; and given antibiotics (which, ironically, made them more vulnerable to disease) to encourage growth as well as ward off other infections. . . . Every condition that predisposed the spread of disease from animal to human actually worsened. Farming became more intensive, slaughtering became more mechanical and faster, products were processed in even more massive lots, and distribution became wider.

Dr. Jeffery Fisher, in his book *The Plague Makers,* takes this further:

> The resistant bacteria that result from this reckless practice do not stay confined to the animals from which they develop. There are no

"cow bacteria" or "pig bacteria" or "chicken bacteria." In terms of the microbial world, we humans along with the rest of the animal kingdom are part of one giant ecosystem. The same resistant bacteria that grow in the intestinal tract of a cow or pig can, and do, eventually end up in our bodies.

The Spread of E. coli–Resistant Strains

Predictably, the agriculture industry has insisted that this is not true, that resistant animal bacteria will not move into the human population. In response, Stuart Levy and a team of research scientists tried an experiment (described in his book *The Antibiotic Paradox*). What they found not only confirmed the movement from farm animal to human but showed even more serious long-term results than expected.

Levy and his team took six groups of chickens and placed them 50 to a cage. Four cages were in a barn; two were just outside. Half the chickens received food containing subtherapeutic doses of oxytetracycline. The feces of all the chickens as well as of the farm family living nearby and farm families in the neighborhood were examined weekly. Within 24 to 36 hours after the chickens had eaten the first batch of antibiotic-containing food, the feces of the dosed chickens showed *E. coli*–resistant bacteria. Soon the undosed chickens also showed *E. coli* resistant to tetracycline. But even more remarkable, by the end of 3 months the *E. coli* of *all* chickens was also resistant to ampicillin, streptomycin, and sulfanamides *even though they had never been fed those drugs*. None of those drugs had been used by anyone in contact with the chickens. Still more startling: At the end of 5 months, the feces of the nearby farm family (who had had no contact with the chickens) contained *E. coli* resistant to tetracycline. By the sixth month, their *E. coli* were also resistant to five other antibiotics. At this point the study ended, noting that none of the families in the neighborhood had any incidence of *E. coli* resistance. However, in a similar but longer study in Germany, it was found that this resistance did move into the surrounding community, taking a little over 2 years.

What is more troubling than this, however, is that *E. coli*, a benign and important symbiotic bacteria found in the gastrointestinal tract of humans and most animals, has been teaching pathogenic bacteria how to resist antibiotics. Even more grim, pathogenic bacteria have been teaching *E. coli* how to become pathogenic. Though there are several *E. coli* that now cause sickness, the most serious is *E. coli* O157:H7, which has caused thousands of illnesses and scores of deaths in the past few years. Because *E. coli* are one of the most pervasive and benign of bacteria (they live in the intestinal systems of most species on this planet), whenever physicians give us (or any animals) antibiotics, the *E. coli* are killed off along with pathogenic bacteria. The massive amounts of antibiotics being used inevitably led to *E. coli* resistance. But because *E. coli* are so important to our health, it was probably crucial that they did. Unfortunately, from one perspective, *E. coli* was a benign bystander that got caught up in our desire to kill off pathogenic bacteria. *E. coli*, in order to survive, chose sides, and has done so with a vengeance. Epidemiologists now feel sure that *E. coli* O157:H7 was taught its virulence by *Shigella* bacteria. Fox, in *Spoiled*, quotes physician and researcher Marguerite Neill who observes that "judicious reflection on the meaning of this finding suggests a larger significance — that *E. coli* O157:H7 is a messenger, bringing an unwelcome message that in mankind's battle to conquer infectious diseases, the opposing army is being replenished with fresh replacements." And these kinds of food-borne diseases are spreading throughout the human food chain.

The Growth of Salmonella

Salmonella in eggs is also a persistent and historically unique problem. Somehow, *Salmonella* bacteria now live in the ovaries of most of the United States chicken stocks. Any eggs they lay are subsequently contaminated. The four common strains of *Salmonella* that transfer from chicken ovaries to their eggs are proving much more resilient than medical researchers expected. As author Nicols Fox relates in her book *Spoiled* all four strains survived refrigeration, boiling, basting with hot oil, and normal "sunny-side-up" frying. The only way to kill the bacterium is to scramble hard at high temperatures, boil for nine minutes or longer, or frying until the yolk is completely hard. Because of this many industry and government representatives are suggesting that all eggs be pasteurized prior to public consumption. Eggs would then come in liquid form in milk-carton-like containers. Because of the contamination Fox believes that we are nearing the end of the shell egg as a staple food for the human species. *Shigella,* a potent dysenteric bacteria, is quite common on vegetable produce, and *Campylobacter* is increasingly found on poultry. As an example of the severity of the problem: In 1946 there were only 723 cases of *Salmonella* food poisoning in the United States. By 1963, there were 18,696. (By contrast, typhoid fever at its worst never exceeded four thousand cases a year.) By 1986, *Salmonella* was estimated to be sickening over 150 thousand people per year. But by far the worst outbreak occurred in 1994, when contaminated Schwan's ice cream alone sickened an estimated 224 thousand people. The same growth patterns are occurring in all other factory farm animal diseases. Estimates from Public Campaign put the total figures for the United Stated to be 9 thousand deaths and 33 million illnesses each year from infected food products. Unlike earlier food-borne diseases, these new "superbugs" can survive the low temperatures of refrigeration or the high temperatures of cooking. Slightly pink hamburger that is infected with *E. coli* can still cause disease; lightly hard-boiled eggs still harbor *Salmonella;* mildly underdone chicken will still sicken the person who eats it with *Campylobacter.* Just as this book was being completed (December 23, 1998) Sarah Lee corporation had to recall $50 to $70 million of meat contaminated with *Listeria* bacteria that had killed and sickened people in nine states. The problem is not uncommon.

United States Department of Agriculture (USDA) baseline estimates in 1995 found 99 percent of all chickens to be contaminated with benign *E. coli* bacteria (a fairly easy bacterium to test for). This is significant because it shows that the meat was being contaminated with the contents of the chicken's gut, something that should not happen during processing. *E. coli* contamination indicates unclean butchering and portends infection by other bacteria that are not benign. Routine inspections after the fact found that from 20 to 80 percent of all chickens, 2 to 29 percent of turkeys, and 49 percent of ground turkey and chicken was contaminated with *Salmonella.* Not only have the bacteria spread, not only have they learned antibiotic resistance, but they are increasingly learning how to survive *environments* that formerly would have killed them (such as hot and cold temperatures). The trend-setter is the dangerous *E. coli* bacteria. *USA Today* reports that it can now live in both orange juice and apple juice, two acidic media that previously killed *E. coli* simply from the amount of acid present.

STAPHYLOCOCCUS AUREUS: THE KING OF RESISTANT BACTERIA

The most alarming of resistant bacteria, in either farm or hospital, has been *Staphylococcus aureus*. Over the past decades, this particular staph species has learned resistance to one antibiotic after another. (Several researchers believe [and have demonstrated *in vitro* to prove their point] that *S. aureus* learned resistance from benign *E. coli* in the human gut.) Not so long ago, staph was still susceptible to two antibiotics: methicillin and vancomycin. Inevitably, methicillin-resistant staph (MRSA) emerged. Physicians and researchers were worried but tried to hold the line, to stop any further adaptation by *S. aureus*. Given the nature of bacteria, they were doomed to failure; on August 2, 1998 *The New York Times* reported the first four world cases of vancomycin-resistant staph. There are *no* antibiotics that can successfully treat vancomycin-resistant *S. aureus*. On December 28, 1998, *USA Today* reported that in response, physicians and hospitals in Washington, D.C., were being urged to severely reduce or cease their use of vancomycin. It is hoped that thereby the bacteria will "forget" how to resist the drug, and it can thus be saved for use to protect the nation's capital in the event of severe epidemic.

Bacteria learn resistance in an inexorable exponential growth curve, and using mathematical modeling researchers had predicted with uncanny accuracy, almost to the month, when vancomycin-resistant staph would appear. It will now proceed into the general population of the world at that same exponential rate. Though scientists hope to stop it, there is in actuality little they can do. Stuart Levy observes that "some analysts warn of present-day scenarios in which infectious antibiotic-resistant bacteria devastate whole human populations."

We do in fact have a serious problem. We have meddled with the microbial world and created bacteria more tenacious and virulent than any known before. They will have effects on both the ecosystem and the human population that can only be guessed at. What is sure, however, is that the antibiotic era is over. The degree and rate of bacterial evolution is so extreme that new antibiotics (of which few are being developed) generate resistance in only a few years instead of the decades that it took previously. It is a frightening future. But there are rays of hope.

WHAT WE CAN DO

If antibiotics are severely curtailed, if they are not used at all in farm production, if they are only used in hospital settings when there is an absolute and verifiable need for them, if general use is strictly confined to cases where there is imminent threat of death or disability, there is every reason to believe that antibiotics can be around for a long time to come. Researchers have found that when bacteria do not encounter antibiotics regularly, they begin to forget how to resist them. A few countries, such as Sweden as Levy notes, that have severely curtailed their antibiotic use have found this to be true in practice as well. A return to farming practices of the past that genuinely care for farm animals and do not treat them like manufacturing units will end the antibiotic resistance problems of factory farming. Keeping the immune system healthy is also important; the human body can fight off most disease if it is well tuned. Finally, the use of herbal alternatives to antibiotics for the treatment of most diseases will ensure that when antibiotics are needed in exceptionally serious conditions, they will still be there.

STEPS TO SLOW DOWN THE EMERGENCE OF ANTIBIOTIC-RESISTANT BACTERIA

1. Take antibiotics only if you really need them.

2. Take them only according to prescription and for as long as the prescription indicates even though you might feel better before then. At this point most of the pathogenic bacteria have been killed (that is why you are feeling better) but there are still small numbers of them that can reproduce again into the billions if you stop the antibiotics. These growing bacteria, because their ancestors were exposed to the antibiotic you are taking, are already learning how to become resistant.

3. Maintain a healthy immune system so that you do not get sick easily.

4. Eat organic foods that have not been exposed to antibiotics.

5. Use herbs as antibiotic alternatives; they do not cause resistance in bacteria.

2

BOTANICAL MEDICINES WITH THE STRONGEST ANTIBIOTIC PROPERTIES

Many herbs have historically been used to treat those infections caused by bacteria that are now antibiotic resistant. Medical research outside the United States has been exploring plants that can treat antibiotic-resistant disease. From before recorded history, plants have been used as the primary healing medicines for human beings. In fact, anthropologists have found medicinal herbs intentionally placed in the grave of a Neanderthal man over 60 thousand years ago. Indigenous cultures throughout the world have long established and highly sophisticated systems of healing using plant medicines. Modern medical researchers have not found anything new, but within their framework they have confirmed the power of plant medicines that have been used for healing for thousands of years.

This research has been sparked in part by a resolution passed by the World Health Organization (WHO) in May 1978. This resolution adopted the contents of a report commissioned by WHO, which noted that for all people to have adequate health care by the year 2000, sources other than Western, technological medicine would have to be used. The report concluded with the recommendation that traditional forms of healing and medicine be pursued to meet the emerging needs of a burgeoning world population.

> As they fell from heaven, the plants said, "Whichever living soul we pervade, that man will suffer no harm."
>
> THE RIG-VEDA

18

WHY BOTANICAL MEDICINES OFFER PROMISE

The research resulting from the resolution adopted by WHO and that engaged in by forward-thinking companies and scientists in Europe and Asia have revealed that instead of being a quaint quackery of our forefathers, many herbs possess strong antibacterial qualities, in many instances being equal to or even surpassing the power of antibiotics. Given the nature of bacteria, it is not unreasonable to assume that new antibiotics would only postpone the problem; bacteria would, in time, become resistant to them. Thus, there is a great deal of promise in addressing this problem through the use of plant medicines instead of antibiotics because plants have a much more complex chemistry than antibiotics. Garlic, for instance, has been found to contain at least 33 sulfur compounds, 17 amino acids, and a dozen other compounds. Pharmaceuticals, in contrast, are usually made from one chemical constituent only. Penicillin is penicillin, tetracycline is tetracycline. Pharmaceutical antibiotics are, in fact, simple substances, not complex, and because of this bacteria can more easily figure out how to counteract their effects. But herbs like garlic are very complex. For instance, yarrow, another healing herb, contains over 120 different compounds that have been identified so far. When a person takes yarrow as herbal medicine they are in actuality taking 120 different medicines into their body and all of these medicines exist in powerful evolutionary balance with each other. They potentiate, enhance, and mitigate each other's effects inside the human body. Faced with this complex chemical makeup, invading

How Complex Is Garlic Compared to Penicillin?

Known active constituents of garlic (there are at least 35 other constituents whose actions are unknown): ajoene, allicin, aliin, allixin, allyl mercaptan, allyl methyl thiosulfinate, allyl methyl trisulfide, allyl propyl disulfide, diallyl disulfide, diallyl hepta sulfide, diallyl hexa sulfide, diallyl penta sulfide, diallyl sulfide, diallyl tetra sulfide, diallyl tri sulfide, dimethyl disulfide, dimethyl trisulfide, dirpopyl disulfide, methyl ajoene, methyl allyl thiosulfinate, propyline sulfide, 2-vinyl-4H-1, 3-tithiin, 3-vinyl-4H-1, 2dithiin, S-allyl cysteine sulfoxide, S-allyl mercapto, cysteine.

Known active constituents of penicillin: penicillin.

bacteria find it much more difficult to develop resistance or avoid the medicine's impact. Perhaps inevitably, scientists are beginning to unconsciously mimic plant medicines. They are finding that combining pharmaceutical antibiotics works better; they are using two and sometimes three antibiotics at once. This is still a long way from the complexity of plant medicines, and this simple mimicry of plant medicines is still not enough; the bacteria notice and develop resistance to the combinations.

TOP 15 ANTIBIOTIC HERBS

The following list is by no means inclusive of all the herbs that are effective for antibacterial-resistant diseases; there are many others. These, however, are arguably among the most powerful and effective. I arrived at this list by using three overlapping criteria: length and type of use in folk medicine, beneficial outcomes in modern clinical practice, and results from modern scientific studies: *in vitro, in vivo,* and in human trials. Thus, these herbs have been found to be powerful healers throughout history, they are noted as reliable healing agents among modern practitioners, and rigorous scientific study has found them to possess potent activity against bacteria. (Information on how to make herbal preparations from these herbs can be found in chapter 4, Making and Using Herbal Medicines. For instance, the tincture formula for echinacea says "Make a 1:5 mixture in 60 proof alcohol." How this and all the other processes are done is explained there.)

For ease of flow in the text, the scientific studies and references for this chapter can be found at the back of the book (see pages 110–126).

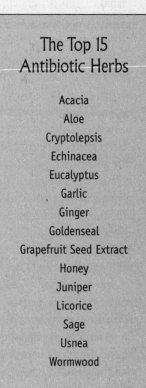

The Top 15 Antibiotic Herbs

Acacia

Aloe

Cryptolepis

Echinacea

Eucalyptus

Garlic

Ginger

Goldenseal

Grapefruit Seed Extract

Honey

Juniper

Licorice

Sage

Usnea

Wormwood

⚘ACACIA (*Acacia* spp.)

Family: Mimosaceae *(Leguminosae).*
Part used: All parts of the plant: flowers, resin, bark, leaf, pods, stems, fruit, spines, root, and root bark.
Collection: The parts of the plant may be gathered at any suitable time of the year: the pods when green, the flowers when in bloom. The roots should be chopped into small sections before drying. The gum may be gathered by breaking off several lower limbs and returning in a few days (or, more traditionally, a line may be cut into the lower part of bark with a sharp hatchet and the gum collected after formation). The collected plant will last quite a long time if well dried, double plastic bagged, and stored in a dark place, off the floor.
Actions: Antimalarial, astringent, antibacterial, antimicrobial, anticatarrhal, hemostatic, anthelmintic, antifungal, mucilaginous (roots and gum), anti-inflammatory, sedative (flowers and leaves).
Active against: *Staphylococcus aureus, Pseudomonas aeruginosa, Salmonella* spp., malaria, *Shigella dysenteriae, Escherichia coli, Proteus mirabilis, Neisseria gonorrhoeae.*

About Acacia

Acacias are quite useful for ulceration in any part of the gastrointestinal tract and for excessive mucus, catarrh, diarrhea, dysentery, gum infection, and hemorrhage. Though rarely used for parasitic infestation in the United States, they are common for that use in other cultures. One species, *Acacia anthelmintica,* is specific for worms in Abyssinia; another, *A. nilotica,* is specific for malaria in Nigeria; and another, *A. polyacantha,* is specific for malaria in Tanzania. They share a common use throughout the world for amebic dysentery.

Acacias, or mimosas as they are sometimes called, grow throughout the temperate world. The United States has several species, *Acacia angustissima* (the only thornless acacia), *A. constricts,* and *A. greggii* being the more common. They grow throughout the southern part of the country as far north as Kansas, from California to Florida. The latter two species are southwestern. Acacia, rarely used now in the United States, continues to be a primary medicinal plant throughout the rest of the world, especially in Asia and Africa. Researchers have noted consistent antibacterial activity by every member of this genus that they have tested. The acacia in some South American cultures has been considered specific (like echinacea) for venomous stings and bites and has been used in much the same manner: the juice of the chewed bark is swallowed, and the chewed bark is placed as a poultice on the bite area. The main species used historically in Western medicine is *A. catechu*. It is a native of India, though it reportedly grows as far west as Jamaica in the Caribbean. The gums of all the acacias are used medicinally, one species, *A. senegal*, being the source of the well-known gum arabic.

A Note on the Use of Acacia

Other than Michael Moore, Western herbalists rarely mention Acacia, and it is seldom used. Acacia's common usage among traditional cultures throughout the world and modern research findings showing its medicinal strength supports a broader use among herbalists everywhere.

Preparation and Dosage

Acacia is generally used as tea, wash, or powder.

Tea: For a strong decoction, use 1 ounce (28 g) of plant material in 16 ounces (475 ml) water, boil for 15 to 30 minutes, let stand overnight, strain.

Use leaves, stems, pods all powdered. Drink 3 to 12 cups a day for shigella, malaria, dysentery, diarrhea. This decoction is both antimicrobial and anti-inflammatory.

Use flowers and leaves as tea for gastrointestinal tract inflammation. Flower tea is sedative.

Use roots to make mucilaginous tea that is antibacterial and anti-inflammatory. Helpful for soothing gastrointestinal tract infections (including mouth and throat), as it coats and soothes, reduces inflammation, and attacks microbial infection.

Wash: *Use tea of leaves, stems, and pods* to wash recent or infected wounds.

Use pods to make wash to treat eyes for conjunctivitis. Add five or six cleaned pods, slightly crushed, to 1 pint (475 ml) water, bring to boil, remove from heat, let steep until it reaches temperature of body heat.

Powder: Leaves, stem, pods, bark, thorns powdered may be applied to fungal infections and infected wounds, and to stop bleeding of wounds and prevent subsequent infection.

Gum preparation: Combine 1 part by weight of acacia gum with 3 parts by volume of distilled water. Place in well-stoppered bottle, shake occasionally, let dissolve, keep refrigerated. (It becomes a slimy goo.) Dosage: 1 to 2 tablespoons (15 to 30 ml) as often as needed for sore inflammations in the gastrointestinal tract from mouth to anus. Especially useful during acute throat infections, ulceration of the mouth, painful gastrointestinal tract from dysenteric disease. The mucilage will coat and soothe and provide antimicrobial action.

Side Effects and Contraindications

None.

Alternatives to Acacia

Mesquite *(Prosopis julifera, P. pubescens)*, a relative and similar-appearing plant with a much broader range in the southwest, may be used identically: same preparation, same dosage, same results.

ALOE *(Aloe vera* and other species)

Family: Liliaceae.
Part used: Usually the fresh juice; in some instances, the dried plant for internal use.
Collection: The fresh plant leaves at any time. The fleshy stems are cut open, and the mucilaginous, jellylike juice, the gel, is used directly on wounds and burns.
Actions: *External use:* antibacterial, antimicrobial, antiviral, wound healing accelerator, anti-inflammatory, antiulcer. *Internal use:* purgative, stimulates smooth muscle contractions.
Active against: *Staphylococcus aureus, Pseudomonas aeruginosa,* herpes simplex 1 and 2.

About Aloe

The first clinical use of penicillin in the United States occurred with the survivors of the Coconut Grove fire in 1942. Burn victims are notoriously prone to severe *Staphylococcus aureus* infections, and before the early sulfa drugs and penicillin, allopathic physicians knew little about how to prevent them. Aloe and honey are perhaps the two most powerful substances that can be applied externally to speed wound healing and prevent infections in burn victims. One especially important attribute possessed by both substances is that they are liquid. They keep burn tissue moist, soothe the damaged tissues, and restore lost body fluids (a problem for burn victims) directly through the skin. At the same time they are potent anti-inflammatories and antibacterials. It is nearly impossible for a staph infection to get started when either substance is used on burned skin. Clinical practitioners who regularly use aloe report excellent results when it is used on skin wounds of any degree of severity and from any source.

Preparation and Dosage

Aloe is very simple to prepare. Just slice or break open the leaves of the fresh plant and apply liberally to any wound or burn until well covered. Use as often as needed for burns of any degree of severity (keeping the burn moist), staph infections of the skin of any degree of severity, and herpes sores.

Side Effects and Contraindications

External Use: none.

Internal Use: hemorrhoids (produces irritation and heat around anus when taken internally), pregnancy (stimulates smooth muscle contractions), active gastrointestinal tract inflammation.

A Note on the Use of Aloe

The dried plant was historically used for constipation in Western medical practice. It is almost never used this way now; the plant is strongly active, with potential unpleasant side effects from internal use, and there are easier alternatives. For burns and infected wounds, aloe and honey are both powerful choices. Several research studies have noted that the fresh aloe juice alone is active; activity declines with time and with any change in color of the juice. The dried plant, with the juice extracted, has been found to be inert against staph bacteria.

Alternatives to Aloe

Honey is one alternative; less desirable choices include echinacea and St. John's wort for wound healing acceleration and to prevent scarring.

CRYPTOLEPSIS (Cryptolepsis sanguinolenta)

Family: Asclepiadaceae.
Part used: The root.
Collection: Cryptolepsis is a twining and scrambling shrub that grows throughout many parts of Africa, primarily along the western coast; the root may be harvested at any time of year.
Actions: Antiparasitic, antimalarial, antibacterial, antifungal.
Active against: Malaria, *Staphylococcus aureus*, *Shigella dysenteriae*, *Neisseria gonorrhea*, *Escherichia coli*, *Candida albicans*, *Campylobacter*, both gram-positive and gram-negative bacteria.

About Cryptolepsis

Cryptolepsis has been used for centuries by traditional African healers in the successful treatment of malaria, fevers, and bloody diarrhea (*sanguinolenta* means "tinged or mixed with blood, bloody"). With the increasing resistance of the malarial parasite to synthetic drugs, medical researchers throughout the world have turned to traditional medicines to find treatment alternatives. Cryptolepsis has been found to be remarkably potent for malaria in human clinical trials. One such trial compared the effectiveness of cryptolepsis with chloroquine, the usual synthetic drug for malaria treatment, in comparative patient populations at the outpatient clinic of the Centre for Scientific Research into Plant Medicine at Mampong-Akwapim in Ghana, West Africa. Clinical symptoms were relieved in 36 hours with cryptolepsis and in 48 hours with chloroquine. Parasitic clearance time was 3.3 days in the patients given cryptolepsis and 2.3 days in the patients given chloroquine — a remarkably comparable time period. Forty percent of the patients using chloroquine reported unpleasant side effects necessitating other medications; those using cryptolepsis reported *no* side effects.

Preparation and Dosage

Cryptolepsis is usually used as a powder or in capsules, tea, or tincture.

External bacterial or fungal infections: Use herb as a finely crushed powder, liberally sprinkled on the site of infection as frequently as needed.

Internal Uses:

Tincture: Make a 1:5 mixture in 60 percent alcohol. Use 20 to 40 drops up to 4 times a day.

Tea: For a preventative tea, combine 1 teaspoon of the herb with 6 ounces (170 ml) of water to make a strong infusion, and take 1 or 2 times a day. For acute conditions, take up to 6 cups (1½ l) a day of the same infusion.

Capsules: As a preventative, take 3 double-ought capsules 2 times a day. In acute conditions, take up to 20 capsules a day.

Dosage for Malaria: 25 milligrams per kilogram (3 pounds) body weight of cryptolepsis extract 3 times daily after meals.

> ### Finding Cryptolepsis
>
> Cryptolepsis is somewhat difficult to obtain in the United States. It can be ordered from Nana Nkatiah (see Resources) or from importers specializing in African herbs.

Side Effects and Contraindications

None noted.

Alternatives to Cryptolepsis

For malaria: *Artemisia annua* or *A. absinthium, Brucea javanica* (fruit, root, or leaf), *Uvaria* spp. (any species, rootbark, stembark, or leaf), garlic vine *(Mansoa standleyi),* or the bark of *Cinchona* spp. from which quinine was made can be used. Though malaria is resistant to quinine, it does not seem to have developed resistance to the more chemically complex *Cinchona* plant itself.

ECHINACEA *(Echinacea angustifolia, E. purpurea)*

Family: Compositae.
Part used: Flower or root.
Collection: For *E. angustifolia:* The root is harvested in either spring or fall. For *E. purpurea:* The flower is harvested after the seeds mature on the cone but while flower petals are still present. The root may also be used.
Actions: Immune stimulant, anti-inflammatory, antibacterial, cell normalizer.
Active against: *Staphylococcus aureus, Streptococcus* spp., mycobacterium (tuberculosis), abnormal cells (direct application necessary).

About Echinacea

Echinacea is without equal in the treatment of three conditions: abnormal Papanicolaou (pap) smear, strep throat, and the very early onset of flus and colds. It is exceptionally useful in two other conditions: as an additive to antibiotic powders and ointments for external application to burns, wounds, and skin infections; and as a wash for poisonous stings and bites.

Abnormal pap smear: Echinacea can easily correct even stage three dysplasia. Whenever echinacea is placed directly on cells that are displaying abnormal properties, the cells tend to return to normal relatively quickly as long as the treatment is assertive and consistent. I have seen no other herb that comes even close to its reliability in this regard.

Strep throat: Direct contact with the tissue at the back of the throat with a tincture of echinacea liberally mixed with saliva is a certain remedy for cases of strep throat. Echinacea actively stimulates saliva and numbs the tissue it comes into contact with, making it perfect for this condition or for any infection causing a sore, swollen throat. I have found this reliably effective, again if treatment is assertive and consistent. In several cases (including a doubting physician), the throat had been positively cultured for *Streptococcus;* healing generally occurs within 24 hours.

Onset of colds and flu: Echinacea should be used at the very early onset of a cold or flu when you feel just the earliest hint of that tingle in the body that signals the approach of symptoms. It is at this point that echinacea is most effective, but it must be taken in large doses and frequently to be effective. When it is taken after the full onset of symptoms, I have found (in over 10 years of clinical experience) that echinacea is not effective, irrespective of its proven ability to increase white blood cell count. Usually, assertive action at this early point in infection will result in averting the full onset of either colds or flu *as long as the immune system is relatively healthy.* A compromised immune system will, after a while, fail to prevent disease in spite of any stimulation you give it (see contraindications, on the next page).

External wounds: Because of its capacity to correct tissue abnormality, echinacea is perfect for this application, and worldwide clinical experience has shown its effectiveness in this area. Echinacea's anti-inflammatory, antibacterial, and cell-normalizing actions all come into powerful play for any external wounds.

Venomous stings and bites: Echinacea has a long history of successful use with venomous stings and bites, from bees to rattlesnakes to scorpions.

Serious blood infections (bacteremia): Though I have not met any modern clinicians who have used echinacea in this most serious of conditions, the eclectic physicians, botanical doctors that practiced in the early part of the twentieth century, used it for this condition, apparently with success. Its proven ability to stimulate white blood cell counts appears to support the use of massive doses for this condition.

Endangered Echinacea

Like goldenseal, echinacea is one of the most overused herbs in the world and is commonly used for conditions that it will not help. As a result, echinacea in the wild is endangered, and whole ecosystems of the herb are being backhoed into oblivion. Unfortunately, *Echinacea angustifolia* is not very easy to grow, though one or two farms produce it in moderate quantities (not enough to meet demand). In my experience, angustifolia root is the herb of choice *only* for abnormal pap smear. The rest of the conditions for which echinacea is indicated can rely on the use of *E. purpurea* blossoms, which naturally renew themselves each year.

Preparation and Dosage

Echinacea may be used as a tincture, tea, powder, poultice, or suppository. To make a tincture, use fresh flowerheads of *E. purpurea* in 1:2 ratio with 95 percent alcohol (for *E. angustifolia* dry root, use 1:5 in 70 percent alcohol).

Internal Uses:

Strep throat: Full dropper (30 drops) of the tincture as often as desired, not less than once each hour until symptoms cease. Mix with saliva and dribble slowly over affected area down back of throat.

Onset of colds and flus: Not less than one dropperful (30 drops) of tincture each hour until symptoms cease. (*Note:* more effective for cold and flu onset in combination with licorice root and red root.)

External Uses:

Venomous stings and bites: Mix alcohol tincture with equal amount of water and wash affected area liberally every 30 minutes.

Wash: Boil 2 ounces (57 g) ground flowerheads or root in 8 ounces (237 ml) water for 15 minutes, let steep 1 hour, strain, and wash wounds and venomous bites and stings liberally as often as needed.

Powder: Powder dried seedheads or root as fine as possible and sprinkle liberally over new or infected wounds. Best in combination with other herbs such as goldenseal, usnea, oak, and wormwood.

Poultice: Mix powder with water until thick, and place it on the affected area.

Suppository for abnormal pap smear: Powder *E. angustifolia* root, mix with vegetable glycerine until the consistency of cookie dough, mix with enough whole wheat flour to make it the consistency of bread dough, shape into suppositories, and freeze. (They will remain pliable but manageable.) Place one suppository each evening (just before sleep) up against the cervix, douche clean the next morning with ½ ounce (15 ml) usnea/calendula tincture in 1 pint (475 ml) water (otherwise the remains will drip out throughout the day). Repeat for 14 days.

Side Effects and Contraindications

Echinacea is a stimulant. Continued immune stimulation in instances of immune depletion to avoid necessary rest or more healthy lifestyle choices will always result in a more severe illness than if the original colds were allowed to progress. Echinacea should not be used if you are getting sick a lot and are using echinacea only to stave off illness without using the time gained to heal the immune system itself through deep healing and recuperation. Rarely, joint pain may occur with large doses taken for extended periods of time.

Alternatives to Echinacea

For immune stimulation at the early onset of colds and flu: cutleaf cone-flower root *(Rudbeckia laciniata* var. *ampla),* wormwood root, balsam root *(Balsamorhiza sagitatta),* boneset *(Eupatorium perfoliatum),* spilanthes spp.

For abnormal pap smear: the root of any other echinacea species and, possibly, calendula (marigold, *Calendula officinalis)* blossoms prepared identically.

For external wounds: usnea, garlic, sage, wormwood, cryptolepsis.

For venomous stings and bites: in descending degree of strength, prickly pear *(Opuntia* spp.) cactus pads. Filet the pad and place on area of bite or sting with gauze bandage, change every 1 to 2 hours; plantain *(Plantago* spp.), chewed leaf of any variety placed on area of bite or wound; tincture or tea wash of cutleaf coneflower root.

EUCALYPTUS *(Eucalyptus* spp.)

Family: Myrtaceae.

Part used: Generally the essential oil, but all parts of the plant, though weaker, are entirely effective.

Collection: The essential oil is commercially produced. A few herbalists are working to reclaim the home production of essential oils, but it is not yet a common practice. However, the essential oil is cheap and is easily found. The plant grows throughout the temperate regions of the world. Native to Australia, it has gone everywhere with humankind. It is overwhelmingly established in California.

The bark and leaves may be harvested at any time they are available. Generally, use the younger, less sickle-shaped leaves and the young branches. Those parts of the tree that have that distinctive eucalyptus odor to the strongest degree is what you are looking for.

Actions: Antibacterial, antimalarial, antifungal, antipyretic, antiseptic, stimulates mucous secretions, diaphoretic.

Active against: Malaria, *Staphylococcus aureus, Shigella dysenteriae, Haemophilus influenzae,* enterobacteria, *Escherichia coli, Pseudomonas aeruginosa, Candida albicans, Klebsiella pneumoniae, Salmonella* spp., *Helicobacter pylori.* The essential oil is effective against just about every microbe.

About Eucalyptus

Eucalyptus is excreted from the body through the lungs and urine. It is therefore especially useful for upper respiratory and urinary tract infections. Test results by researchers throughout the world have confirmed eucalyptus as one of the agents with the broadest spectrum against antibiotic-resistant disease. Though there has been a great deal of research on its effects in animals, there has been little in humans other than its long historical use by indigenous peoples and, subsequently, medical practitioners of many countries. One major advantage of the herb and essential oil is that its scent is pleasing, especially in a sickroom and to the sick. This uplifting odor of the herb is in its own way a powerful additive to the healing process in that it helps alleviate the inevitable depression attending long and severe illness.

Preparation and Dosage

The leaf can be prepared as tea, powder, tincture, gargle, nasal spray, steam inhalant, smoke, or douche. The essential oil is used as an inhalant for aromatherapy.

Tea: 1 ounce (25 g) herb in 8 ounces (237 ml) water, steep 30 minutes. Use as external wash for infected wounds or up to 6 times a day internally for colds, sore throat, bronchial congestion, fevers, chills.

Antimalarial Properties

Note: Though I have been unable to find any clinical trial data for the use of eucalyptus as an antimalarial agent, it has been found specific (and powerful) for that microbial disease in several *in vitro* studies. Historical use, both in indigenous practice and in medicine, shows it to be specific as a treatment for malaria as well as typhoid, diphtheria, and influenza, especially with attending fetid conditions such as upper respiratory infection with foul breath or fetid catarrh, infected wound with foul discharge, foul diarrhea, vaginal infection with foul discharge, and gangrenous conditions.

Powder: Dust on infected skin, wounds, ulcerations as needed.

Tincture: Fresh herb 1:2 with 95 percent alcohol, dried herb 1:5 in 65 percent alcohol; 10 to 30 drops in water for same conditions as tea.

Gargle: 30 drops tincture in 6 ounces (177 ml) water, gargle up to 3 times a day, and swallow.

Nasal spray: 30 drops of tincture (or 5 drops essential oil) in 1 ounce (30 ml) water as nasal spray as often as desired.

Steam: Boil 3 to 4 ounces (75 to 100 g) of herb in 1 gallon (4 l) water, remove from heat, and inhale steam.

Smoke: In sweat lodge or sauna, or in rolled cigarettes for upper respiratory conditions.

Douche: 2 drams (8 ml) tincture to 1 pint (475 ml) water once daily.

Essential oil: 10 drops in hot water in narrow-necked vessel, and the resulting vapor inhaled. In a diffuser daily, or diluted in the bath during illness.

Side Effects and Contraindications

The eucalyptus oil begins to be toxic if taken internally in any quantity over 4 or 5 drops. The oil can be irritating when directly placed on the skin. Ingestion of too much tea can result in intestinal cramping.

Alternatives to Eucalyptus

For fetid conditions: alder (*Alnus* spp.) bark
For internal antibacterial actions: garlic
As essential oil: tea tree oil

Recent clinical research has shown tea tree oil to be specifically active against antibiotic-resistant disease organisms. Other essential oils showing exceptional antibiotic activity are rosemary, yarrow, wormwood, grapefruit seed, thyme, and feverfew. A recent study reported at a meeting of the American Society of Microbiology noted that essential oils are extremely powerful in the treatment of pneumonia. Lead researcher Diane Horne noted that the essential oils of thyme, rosewood, and oregano cause pneumonia-causing antibiotic-resistant bacteria to simply "go to pieces."

✿GARLIC (Allium sativum)

Family: Liliaceae.
Part used: The bulb and cloves are used for medicine and food.
Collection: The plant is indigenous to Asia but is now grown throughout the world. The bulb is harvested in early fall when the leaves begin to wither.
Actions: Antibacterial, antiviral, antiseptic, antiparasitic, antiprotozoan, antiviral, antifungal, anthelmintic, immune-stimulating, hypotensive, diaphoretic, antispasmodic, cholagogue.
Active against: Tuberculosis, *Shigella dysenteriae*, *Staphylococcus aureus*, *Pseudomonas aeruginosa*, *Candida albicans*, *Escherichia coli*, *Streptococcus* spp., *Salmonella* spp., *Campylobacter* spp., *Proteus mirabilis*, herpes simplex, influenza B, HIV, and many others. Both gram-positive and gram-negative bacteria.

About Garlic

Garlic, a well-known culinary herb, is thought to have originated in the high plains of west central Asia and has been used medicinally for some five thousand years. This is the most powerful herb for the treatment of antibiotic-resistant disease (followed by grapefruit seed extract). No other herb comes close to the multiple system actions of garlic, its antibiotic activity, and its immune-potentiating power.

When the bulb is bruised or crushed, garlic produces a byproduct compound called allicin. The odorless, sulfur-containing amino acid in garlic, alliin, comes into contact with an enzyme, allinase, and produces a conversion to allicin, which is the primary compound responsible for garlic's strong odor. Allicin, diallyl disulfide, diallyl trisulfide, ajoene (the combination of allicin and diallyl disulfide), and several additional compounds in garlic have all shown antibiotic activity. Extracts made from the whole clove of garlic or separate individual compounds have consistently shown a broad-spectrum antibiotic range effective against both gram-negative and gram-positive bacteria and most major infectious bacteria. Garlic juice diluted to as little as one part in 125,000 has been found to inhibit the growth of bacteria. Clinical studies, such as one in 1984 by Singh and Shukla, have repeatedly shown that garlic is active against strains of bacteria that are highly resistant to antibiotics. Unlike many herbs, garlic is directly effective against viruses. Garlic is perhaps the most extensively tested herb in the world; *in vitro, in vivo,* and human trials have shown its powerful effectiveness against bacterial and viral infectious agents.

For stimulating immune function and for lowering blood pressure and cholesterol counts, garlic works well either raw, cooked, or encapsulated. For treating active bacterial infection, it should be consumed either in uncooked whole form or as juice.

Controlling Garlic Odor

The difficulty with garlic is, of course, its strong odor, and many people are uncomfortable using it for this reason. Deodorized garlic capsules are now available through many health food stores.

Raw garlic or its juice kills bacterial infection in the gastrointestinal tract as soon as it comes into direct contact with the organisms. When used as a douche, the garlic juice (or even a garlic clove inserted in the vagina) will kill bacterial infection. When used in nose drops, the garlic covers the surface of the nasal passages and sinuses and kills off infection there. When used on athlete's foot and surface skin infections, its action is sure and rapid.

In just a few of the many trials, researchers have used garlic in both humans and animals to successfully treat the four strains of bacteria that cause most of the world's dysentery. Chinese physicians have found garlic exceptionally effective against cryptococcal meningitis and viral encephalitis. African physicians have used it as primary medicine successfully against amebic dysentery, toxoplasmosis, *Cryptosporidium* spp., and *pneumocystis* spp. American researchers have shown that garlic activates the immune system to help protect the body from infection and, when infection occurs, to stimulate the immune system to attack invading bacteria more effectively. Beyond these potent actions, garlic has also shown repeatable and impressive clinical results in the treatment of heart disease, high blood pressure, high cholesterol, cancer, stress, fatigue, and aging.

If only one herb could be used to combat an epidemic spread of antibiotic-resistant bacteria, this would be it.

Preparation and Dosage

May be taken fresh (as juice or as cloves), in capsules, as tincture, or in food.

Fresh cloves: Eat 1 clove up to 3 times a day for prevention. The cloves may be diced and mixed with honey for palatabilty and to reduce nausea. During acute episodes, 3 to 9 *bulbs* a day are reportedly being used by some clinicians. (They report that the best way is to juice the bulbs and drink with carrot or tomato juice. *Caution:* See Side Effects and Contraindications.)

Fresh juice: Juice the bulbs as needed; take ¼ to 1 teaspoon (1 to 5 ml) as needed.

Capsules: 3 capsules 3 times a day as preventative. During acute episodes: up to 30 capsules a day.

Tincture: Fresh bulb 1:2, in 95 percent alcohol, 40 drops up to 6 times a day.

Food: Lots in everything. Increase during acute episodes.

Side Effects and Contraindications

Nausea, vomiting. Many practitioners believe that garlic is most effective as an antibiotic when used fresh, either raw or as juice. Garlic is, unfortunately, exceptionally pungent and acrid in any quantity as a raw herb or as juice. Care should be taken in consuming it in quantity. Though an entire bulb produces little juice, it is exceptionally potent and is, actually, quite a strong emetic even in small quantities. The best approach is to start with ¼ teaspoon (1 ml) in a full glass of something like tomato or carrot juice and work up from there. The juice from one bulb of garlic combined with even 24 ounces (710 ml) of carrot juice causes, at least in me, almost immediate vomiting. From this rather unpleasant beginning I found that frequent doses, from ¼ to 1 teaspoon (1 to 5 ml) in 16 ounces (473 ml) of carrier (tomato juice is pretty good) each hour is a good way to get a large quantity of garlic juice into the system. Caution must be exercised; the quantities used should be small and increased only as the body shows no signs of adverse reactions. You won't die if you take too much, but you will want to. When you finally do vomit, it will be with exceptional vigor. A growing number of practitioners feel that garlic in capsule form is as effective as fresh or juiced cloves.

Garlic is not suggested for nursing mothers, as it affects the taste of the milk and may interfere with nursing. It is excreted from the body through the lungs; this may irritate loved ones and strangers alike.

Alternatives to Garlic

Wild garlics, onions (though weaker they possess many of the same actions), and (within a certain range) grapefruit seed extract (see individual entry).

GINGER *(Zingiber officinale)*

Family: Zingiberaceae.
Part used: The root is used for medicine and food.
Collection: The plant is indigenous to Asia but is now grown throughout the world. The root is harvested in the fall when the leaves and stem have begun to dry.
Actions: Antibacterial, antiviral, circulatory stimulant, anti-inflammatory, diaphoretic, antispasmodic, antiemetic, antifungal, hypotensive, anticlotting agent, carminative, antiarthritic, analgesic, antitussive.
Active against: Malaria, *Shigella dysenteriae, Staphylococcus aureus, Pseudomonas aeruginosa, Candida albicans, Escherichia coli, Klebsiella pneumoniae, Streptococcus* spp., *Salmonella* spp.

About Ginger

Ginger has a long historical tradition in warm climates as a food additive. Like many other spices used on food, it possesses strong antibacterial activity against several food-borne pathogens, especially three of those now plaguing commercial foods: *Shigella, E. coli,* and *Salmonella.* Ginger is also active against many human pathogenic bacteria.

It has traditionally been a primary herb of choice for treating colds and flu. It is especially useful for children in that it is safe in large quantities and yet tastes quite good. A relatively unknown fact is that ginger's antitussive (anticough) action rivals that of codeine, and its strong expectorant and antihistamine actions help thin bronchial mucus and move it up and out of the system. This makes it a perfect herb for upper respiratory infections. Ginger relieves pain, stimulates immune activity, reduces inflammation, and stimulates sweating, thus helping lower fevers.

Like many traditional fever herbs, it is specific against malaria. It is anticramping and reduces or eliminates diarrhea, making it highly useful for dysentery. It is an antinausea herb, helping to prevent vomiting. Since it stimulates peripheral circulation, it is warming to the extremities and helps prevent the kinds of chills associated with malaria, colds, and flus.

One of its clinical uses is for burns. The juice of fresh ginger, soaked into a cotton ball and applied to burns, acts as an immediate pain reliever (even on open blisters), reduces blistering and inflammation, and provides antibacterial protection against infection.

> ## Enjoying Ginger
>
> Two of the best ways to take ginger as food are pickled ginger, often served along with sushi in Japanese restaurants, and candied ginger root slices. Both make great snacks, can be eaten in large quantities, and are a healthy stimulant for the system.

It has a wide range of action in the human body, having been found effective in the treatment of cataracts, heart disease, migraines, stroke, amenorrhea, angina, athlete's foot, bursitis, chronic fatigue, colds and flu, coughs, depression, dizziness, fever, infertility, erection problems, kidney stones, Raynaud's disease, sciatica, tendinitis, and viral infections.

Preparation and Dosage

May be taken as tea, in capsules, as tincture, or in food.

Tea: Fresh root — 1 ounce (25 g) steeped for 5 minutes in 8 ounces (237 ml) water. Dried root — 1½ teaspoons in 8 ounces (237 ml) water, simmered for 10 minutes. During acute episodes, drink throughout the day.

Capsules: Grind herb to powder and encapsulate; take 3 capsules 3 times a day as stimulant to circulatory and immune systems. During acute episodes, take up to 25 capsules a day.

Tincture: Fresh root 1:2 with 95 percent alcohol, 10 to 20 drops up to 4 times a day. Dried root (not as good) 1:5 in 60 percent alcohol, 20 to 40 drops up to 4 times a day.

Food: In everything and anything, often.

Side Effects and Contraindications

Avoid large doses during pregnancy.

Alternatives to Ginger

Alpinia (little ginger, *Alpinia galanga*), garlic, onions, horseradish, mustard.

GOLDENSEAL *(Hydrastis canadensis)*

Family: Ranunculaceae.
Part used: Roots and leaves.
Collection: The roots should be harvested in the fall after the seeds have ripened. Only plants 3 years old or older should be taken (see box: Help Protect Endangered Goldenseal on page 41). The above-ground plant can be harvested at any time.
Actions: Antiseptic, antibacterial, antihemorrhagic, antifungal, antiamebic, astringent, expectorant, diaphoretic, mucosal anti-inflammatory, mucosal stimulant, mucosal tonic, antitumor (cytotoxic).
Active against: *Staphylococcus aureus* (whole herb). A primary constituent of goldenseal, berberine, has been found active *in vitro* against *Vibrio cholerae, Streptococcus, pyogenes, Shigella* spp., *Candida albicans, Escherichia coli, Klebsiella pneumoniae, Salmonella typhimurium* and *S. paratyphi, Corynebacterium diphtheriae*, tuberculosis, *Giardia lamblia,* and *Trichomonas vaginalis,* among many others.

About Goldenseal

With this herb, more than any other, it is possible to find completely conflicting perspectives from clinicians of equal stature and length of practice. Some clinicians consider it to be a reliable immune stimulant, antibiotic, and antiviral. Many others do not. All can cite impressive clinical experience. In fact, very little research has been done on goldenseal, and almost no human clinical trials have been conducted. The science has generally focused on one constituent of goldenseal: berberine. Here, too, the controversy continues. Goldenseal has another major constituent: hydrastine. Some researchers consider this constituent to be the active one; others, the berberine. All note extensive data to support their positions. Furthermore, several respected clinical herbalists support the use of massive doses of goldenseal for systemic bacterial infections, whereas others think only tiny amounts should be used. Both sides cite long-term clinical experience to support their positions.

One Seattle clinician notes that he has worked with severe mucous membrane infections in AIDS patients for the past 20 years and that the incidence of antibiotic-resistant disease in this population has grown. Dosages of goldenseal that were effective 12 years ago (10 capsules per day) are no longer sufficient, and the dose range has now risen to 25 capsules per day to combat active bacterial and fungal infections in the body's mucosal systems. This same clinician has found goldenseal effective as a systemic antibacterial agent and has successfully used it for treatment of a medically cultured antibiotic-resistant staph infection in the foot that had not responded to any antibiotics. With conventional medical treatment, the foot would have been amputated. The dosage in this case was 25 double-ought capsules a day for 2 weeks.

Other clinicians insist that side effects such as excessive drying of the membrane systems, severe abdominal cramping, vomiting, possible liver damage, and nervous tremors will occur with doses that large and that in any event, the dose will not be effective. Clinicians who use high doses deny ever having seen such symptoms in their patients even with decades of experience at such dose levels. A monkey wrench for the low-dose purists: lengthy historical use, Food and Drug Administration (FDA) reports (notoriously overresponsive to even a whiff of adverse reactions), and poison center reports all fail to note the side effects ascribed to high doses of goldenseal. A clear resolution of the conflicting positions remains elusive. One factor that might be important: In traditional Chinese medicine goldenseal relatives (such as *Coptis chinensis*) are considered to be contraindicated for people that tend to be dry and thin. It is generally used for people who are considered moist — i.e., moist skin and slightly plump. It might be that people with more naturally occurring body moisture have less tendency for their mucous membranes to "dry out" when they take goldenseal or its analogues.

When taken internally the herb does not appear to simulate the immune system directly but rather the healthy functioning of the mucous membranes of the body and, as a result, the level of active immunoglobulin A antibodies (IgA) in the mucus. IgA is one of the antibodies in the human body, and it infuses the mucous membranes in order to fight infections that seek to gain a toehold there. Stimulation of the mucous membranes and the IgA antibodies then helps prevent infections. Effective functioning or even proper stimulation of the mucous membranes through the use of goldenseal has been shown in one clinical trial to combat a viral infection more effectively than pharmaceutical drugs. In this case it was a severe infection of the eye with *Chlamydia trachomatis,* a common disease in the Third World. For the *Chlamydia* infection, the eye drops described below were used daily for 3 weeks. For colds and flu, goldenseal seems most effective when used in the later stages of a cold when there is active infection of the mucous membranes. As a general tonic for colds and flu, it would be effective only in small doses if the mucosal system is not functioning properly. Otherwise it is not indicated.

Goldenseal is also excreted in the urine and so can directly combat infection in the urinary tract, although many other herbs, such as uva ursi, are cheaper and as effective for that system.

Clinical trials have shown its reliable effectiveness in combatting dysentery-type diseases. Empiric clinicians also report success in this area, one clinician in Boulder using it successfully with the particularly virulent food-borne *E. coli* O157:H7, which causes bloody diarrhea. In this instance, the *E. coli* infection, from contaminated apple juice, was treated by the use of three berberine-containing herbs (goldenseal, barberry, and Oregon grape root) in an equal-parts tincture combination: 20 drops in water every 2 or 3 hours. All bleeding stopped within 24 hours.

Goldenseal seems best when used for six purposes: for active infections, inflammations, or ulcerations in the gastrointestinal tract, from gums to rectum; for active infections in the sinuses when used as snuff or sinus wash; for active infections in the vagina when used as a douche; for active skin infections when used as a powder or wash; for active eye infections when used as a wash; and as a stimulant/tonic (when used in moderation and for limited duration) in general for mucous membranes throughout the body to help tone them and help them serve their function as one of the first lines of defense against bacterial infection.

Clinical (human) trials using berberine sulfate, a derived constituent of goldenseal, have shown dependable effectiveness, surpassing pharmaceuticals, against diarrhea caused by enterotoxigenic *E. coli*. Berberine sulfate has been shown to significantly inhibit the intestinal secretory response induced by both cholera and *E. coli* infection *in vivo*.

Goldenseal is extensively overused, often for inappropriate conditions. The best results can be obtained if you focus on using the herb for the conditions described here, begin with minimum doses, and work up.

Preparation and Dosage

As a powder for topical application, douche, tincture, in capsules, as a snuff.

Powder may be applied to any cuts, scrapes, or infected wounds, especially those caused by *Staphylococcus* organisms.

Douche: 1 teaspoon (5 ml) of powdered root infused in 1 pint (475 ml) of water, the liquid used each morning and evening until symptoms abate (as an alternative, ⅓ ounce [10 ml] of tincture in 1 pint [475 ml] of water).

Tincture: Fresh herb, 1:2 in 90 percent alcohol, 15 to 30 drops up to 4 times a day; dry herb, 1:5 with 60 percent alcohol, 30 to 75 drops up to 4 times a day; dry root, 1:5 in 70 percent alcohol, 20 to 50 drops up to 4 times a day. As capsules: Double-ought capsules, 1 to 2 capsules up to 4 times a day. In some acute conditions: up to 25 capsules a day for as long as 10 days.

Infusion: For viral or bacterial eye infections an infusion of the powdered root, 1 teaspoon in 6 ounces (177 ml) hot water, steeped 1 hour, and used as eye drops.

Snuff: Place two thin lines of root powder on a table and sniff them vigorously, each line into a different nostril, up to 3 times a day for up to 7 days.

Help Protect Endangered Goldenseal

Goldenseal is extremely expensive and is rarely indicated. Use alternatives when possible, as it is an endangered plant because of overuse. When possible, you should use organically grown roots and *never* harvest the wild populations unless you are the caretaker of a large population and can reliably harvest for your community's use without endangering the plant population's survival. Though some herbalists insist it's not true, laboratory study shows that the herb, though weaker than the root, may be used interchangeably with the root for medicine, and this is encouraged to protect plant populations in the wild. The above-ground plant is used throughout the Caribbean and in Europe as tea for medicinal use.

Side Effects and Contraindications

Do not use during pregnancy. Some clinicians report abdominal cramping, nervous tremors, and excessive drying of the mucous membranes when large doses are used.

Alternatives to Goldenseal

Probably the closest herb to goldenseal is goldthread, *Coptis* spp. The Chinese species, *Coptis chinensis,* has a root larger than goldenseal; the American species, *Coptis trifoliata,* has a tiny threadlike root system, and it takes a great deal of it to make sufficient medicine. However, they are used almost identically. Laboratory study verifies their actions against antibiotic-resistant bacteria, and their historical use indicates that they are an efficient substitute for goldenseal. One species in India, *C. teeta,* has been traditionally used as an effective anti-malarial herb and it has been verified *in vitro* to be active against the malarial parasite.

Other substitutes for specific uses include:

Mucous membrane tonic: yerba manza *(Anemopsis californica).*

Topical infections: usnea, coptis, Oregon grape root *(Mahonia* spp.), barberry *(Berberis vulgaris).*

Eye wash: Oregon grape/usnea/rose hip; equal parts, infused in water.

Vaginal douche: usnea/calendula tincture; equal parts, in 1 pint water.

Gum infections: elephant tree *(Bursera microphylla)* or myrrh *(Comiphora* spp.), oak bark or rhatany *(Krameria* spp.) tinctures in combination.

Intestinal infections with diarrhea: cryptolepsis or artemisia combined with either oak bark or rhatany.

Snuff: skunk cabbage *(Lysichiton* spp. or *Lysichitum* spp. or *Symplocarpus foetidus),* Oregon grape, barberry, coptis.

GRAPEFRUIT SEED EXTRACT (GSE) *(Citrus paradisi)*

Family: Rutaceae.

Part used: Seed and fruit peel, although there is evidence that the leaves are equally effective (see comment under Preparation and Dosage).

Collection: The seed and peel from the fresh ripe fruit (see comment under Preparation and Dosage); the leaves at any time.

Actions: Antibacterial, antimicrobial, antiseptic, antiviral, antifungal, anthelmintic, antiparasitic. Of all herbs, it is perhaps the only true "antibiotic," the literal meaning of which is "antilife."

Active against: GSE is active against a very large number of microorganisms. Most studies on GSE have been *in vitro*, that is, in laboratory trials, *not* with human beings. *In vitro* activity is not always a reliable indicator of *in vivo* action by herbal medicines. There have been few clinical trials using GSE that I have been able to find. However, GSE *has* been found to be effective in cleaning hospital equipment, swimming pools, drinking water supplies, and in veterinary practice. I have used it effectively in treatment of *Helicobacter pylori*, the organism that causes stomach ulceration. A brief listing of activity (by organism and disease; generally GSE is active against multiple species and strains): *Shigella, Staphylococcus, Pseudomonas aeruginosa, Giardia lamblia, Diplococcus pneumoniae, Haemophilus influenzae, Mycobacterium* spp. (causing tuberculosis), *Campylobacter, Candida albicans, Escherichia coli, Streptococcus, Salmonella, Klebsiella, Proteus, Cholera, Chlamydia trachomatis, Trichomonas vaginalis, Legionella pneumoniae, Helicobacter pylori,* herpes simplex 1, influenza A2, measles, and many others, including both gram-positive and gram-negative bacteria. One study showed that of 794 bacterial strains and 93 fungal strains, a commercial preparation of grapefruit seed extract was effective against 249 *Staphylococcus* species and *S. aureus* strains, 86 *Streptococcus* species, 232 enterococcus species, 77 *Enterobacter* species, 86 *E. coli* strains, 22 *Klebsiella* species, 18 *Proteus* species, 77 yeast fungi, and 22 mold fungi strains.

About Grapefruit Seed Extract

Grapefruit seed extract (GSE) and garlic are the two most powerful broad-spectrum antibiotics available for use. In descending degrees of potency, they are followed by eucalyptus, juniper, usnea, cryptolepsis, and wormwood. GSE also has broad-spectrum activity against yeasts, fungi, and many other organisms, surpassing garlic's range by a considerable margin. Furthermore, the broad activity of GSE is available from minute doses of the extract, whereas garlic must be taken in relatively large doses to be equivalently effective as a straight antibiotic.

GSE is becoming more and more common in industrial applications as an environmentally friendly cleanser and antiseptic. It can sterilize cooking pots, surgical instruments — nearly anything. There are two clear negatives: GSE can kill off intestinal or skin bacteria where garlic will not, whatever the amount consumed, and GSE is much more difficult to make at home. It must be either purchased or made from plants with a limited range of growth. Garlic may be grown easily throughout most of North America and the world. An additional strength of garlic is that it adds considerable health-supporting and immune-enhancing benefits, a range of action not achievable from GSE at all. One particular strength of GSE over garlic is its use as a disinfectant. GSE has been found to be more powerful as a cleaning disinfectant than standard hospital preparations. One study showed it to be 100 percent effective, versus 98 percent for commercial hospital preparations and 72 percent for rubbing alcohol. Perhaps the best listing of the many laboratory studies on GSE is contained in Shalila Sharamon and Bodo Baginski's *The Healing Power of Grapefruit Seed* from Lotus Light Publishing (1996).

Preparation and Dosage

Use as diluted extract for internal use, as douche, as wash, as nasal spray, as water purifier when traveling in foreign countries or to treat water-borne infectious disease, as disinfectant for sickrooms, medical instruments, hands.

Fresh leaves, seed, and fruit peel: Generally, GSE is professionally manufactured. The exact manufacturing process is a closely kept secret, and there is some (disputed) evidence that the commercial process involves more than a simple extraction procedure. It is unknown whether simple home extraction processes will produce the same efficacy as the commercial extract. The seeds, peel, and leaves may all be used.

Seeds only: To prepare the closest thing to the commercial preparation, use seeds only. Grind well. Add enough 95 percent grain alcohol to moisten well without the mixture being soupy. It should look like damp sawdust. Let stand for 24 hours, covered. Add 70 percent vegetable glycerine and 30 percent spring or distilled water in a 1:3 ratio.

Specifically, if you have 10 ounces (284 g) grapefruit seeds, then you need 30 ounces (887 ml) liquid, of which 21 ounces (621 ml) will be vegetable glycerine and 9 ounces (266 ml) will be water. Add the liquid to the grapefruit seed and alcohol mixture, mix well, and let stand for 2 weeks. Decant, press the pulp well to extract any remaining moisture, and store in amber bottles out of the sun. This will produce an extract similar in taste and texture to a commercial preparation; however, I have been unable to determine whether it will have the same antibacterial activities as a commercial extract. All human dosages were developed from trial with the commercial extract, as were all antibacterial studies.

Note: GSE is extremely bitter. Nothing will mask its bitterness except citrus fruit drinks such as orange and grapefruit juice, lemonade, and limeade. As few as 5 drops in a 12-ounce (355 ml) glass of apple juice is unpleasantly bitter.

Commercial extract dosages: Extensive animal treatment has shown that high levels can be tolerated in the treatment of acute disease in farm stock. The usual dosage for humans is much smaller.

Animal dosages: Many animal trials have shown that in the treatment of diseases caused by viruses, parasites, bacteria, and fungi; 1 drop of extract per 2 pounds (1 kg) of body weight may be used. This amount is increased in especially acute conditions.

Internal use (human): 3 to 15 drops in citrus juice 2 to 3 times a day. In any disease condition, the minimum should be used and the dose only

Citrus Oil Antibacterial Activity

Though it has proved impossible to discover the process used to make commercial GSE, there is significant evidence that the grapefruit plant and all the citrus family possess potent antibacterial activity. A cursory reading of the literature shows reliable activity against *Staphylococcus, Salmonella, Pseudomonas,* and *Shigella* organisms from grapefruit, lemon, and lime: peel, seed, leaf, and essential oil. One of the most potent essential oils, used for broad-spectrum antibiotic action, is *Citrus bergamia.* (Called bergamot in common use, it is often confused with plants of the *Monarda* species.) The essential oils from citrus species are generally made from the peel or rinds of the fruit. All have shown strong antibacterial activity. The peels have historically been used as medicine throughout the world, in many instances for bacterial and amebic diseases.

increased if no adverse reactions occur. The possible side effects and contraindications should be kept in mind.

Douche: 6 to 12 drops in 1 pint (475 ml) water 2 times a day for up to 1 week.

Nasal spray: 3 to 5 drops in nasal spray bottle up to 6 times a day.

Wash: 20 to 40 drops in 1 pint (475 ml) water for infected wounds.

Diarrhea or dysentery preventative: 3 drops per day when traveling.

To purify water: 3 drops per 8 ounces (237 ml) water (or 350 gallons [906 l] per 1 million gallons [3,785,400 l] for municipal water supply).

Disinfectant: 30 to 40 drops per 1 quart (1 l) water. Use to clean hands, surgical instruments, rooms, linens.

For bandages: 30 to 40 drops in 1 quart (1 l) distilled water in spray bottle; spray on bandages before use.

Side Effects and Contraindications

GSE must be diluted before use. Excessive internal doses over extended periods can kill off all intestinal bacteria much as broad-spectrum antibiotics will, with the same problematic side effects. The undiluted extract can cause skin and mucous membrane irritation. The extract will cause severe eye irritation. Generally, the extract should always be used diluted and not used for eye infections. Keep it out of the reach of children. Caution is indicated in pregnancy. If it is used for serious bacterial infection to the extent that intestinal bacteria are killed off, the gut should be repopulated as soon as possible. Yogurt and acidophilus are recommended for this purpose.

Alternatives to Grapefruit Seed Extract

Garlic. All citrus species, which have shown remarkable antibiotic activity in both traditional use and scientific study. The most powerful appear to be *Citrus bergamia, C. limetta, C. limon, C. aurantiifolia, C. grandis, C. reticulata,* and *C. sinensis.*

⊕HONEY (concentrated nectar of wildflowers of various species)

Part used: The honey syrup itself.
Collection: In the fall from beehives.
Actions: Antibiotic, antiviral, anti-inflammatory, anticarcinogenic, expectorant, antiallergenic, laxative, antianemic, tonic, antifungal, immune stimulant, cell regenerator.
Active against: *Staphylococcus aureus*, *Streptococcus* spp., enterococcus, *Helicobacter pylori*.

About Honey

Honey is the nectar of the flowers of plants, gathered by the bee, stored in its stomach for transport to the hive, and there concentrated by evaporation. Natural honeys are from a profusion of wildflowers, whatever grows locally. Natural honeys, unlike the alfalfa or clover honeys of today, are rarely gathered from a single species unless that plant species exists in great abundance (as heather does in Scotland). Natural bee honeys therefore possess the essence of a multitude of wild plants, all of them medicinal. Honeybees find a great attraction for many strongly medicinal plants: vitex, jojoba, elder, toadflax, balsam root, echinacea, valerian, dandelion, wild geranium — in fact, almost any flowering medicinal herb, as well as the more commonly known alfalfas and clovers. The nectar from many medicinal plants is present in any wildflower honey mix. In addition to the plant's medicinal qualities, the plant nectars are subtly altered, in ways that modern science has been unable to explain, by their brief transport in the bees' digestive system. Before regurgitation, the nectars combine in unique ways with the bees' digestive enzymes to produce new compounds.

Honey, often insisted to be just another simple carbohydrate (like white sugar), actually contains, among other things, a complex assortment of enzymes, organic acids, esters, antibiotic agents, trace minerals, proteins, carbohydrates, hormones, and antimicrobial compounds. One pound of the average honey contains 1333 calories (compared with white sugar at 1748 calories), 1.4 grams of protein, 23 milligrams of calcium, 73 milligrams of phosphorus, 4.1 milligrams of iron, 1 milligram of niacin, and 16 milligrams of vitamin C, and vitamin A, beta carotene, the complete complex of B vitamins, vitamin D, vitamin E, vitamin K, magnesium, sulfur, chlorine, potassium, iodine, sodium, copper, manganese, high concentrations of hydrogen peroxide, and formic acid. Honey, in fact, contains more than 75 different compounds. Many of the remaining substances in honey are so complex (4 to 7 percent of the honey) that they have yet to be identified.

Honey as a consistent additive to food has shown remarkable results in medical trials. Of one group of 58 boys, 29 were given 2 tablespoons (30 ml) of honey each day (one in the morning and one in the evening), and the other 29 boys were given none. All received the same diet, exercise, and rest. All were of the same age and general health. After one year, the boys receiving honey showed an 8½ percent increase in hemoglobin and an overall increase in vitality, energy, and general appearance over the other boys.

Honey has been effectively used clinically for the treatment of fist-sized ulcers extending to the bone and for third-degree burns. Complete healing has consistently been reported without the need for skin grafts and with no infection or muscle loss. Additionally, honey has outperformed antibiotics in the treatment of stomach ulceration, gangrene, surgical wound infections, surgical incisions, and the protection of skin grafts, corneas, blood vessels, and bones during storage and shipment.

Honey is also exceptionally effective in respiratory ailments. A Bulgarian study of 17,862 patients found that honey was effective in improving chronic bronchitis, asthmatic bronchitis, bronchial asthma, chronic and allergic rhinitis, and sinusitis. It is effective in the treatment of colds, flu, respiratory infections, and general depressed immune problems.

Why Wildflower Honey Only?

Wildflower honey should be used, not the clover or alfalfa honey readily available in grocery stores. Alfalfa and clover crops are heavily sprayed with pesticides and do not have the broad activity available in multiple-plant honeys. Furthermore, large commercial honey growers may often supplement their bees' food with sugar water, which dilutes the honey's power. Pure wildflower honey should lightly burn or sting the back of the throat when taken undiluted.

Preparation and Dosage

Direct application to wounds or internal use for immune stimulation, overall health improvement, treatment of colds, flus, and respiratory infections.

External Uses:
Burns (first, second, and third degree): Apply directly at full strength, cover by sterile bandage, change daily.
Ulceration, bed sores (even to the bone): Same as above.
Impetigo: Same as above.
Infected wounds: Same as above.
Wounds: Same as above.

Internal Uses:
Undiluted: As a preventative, take 1 tablespoon (45 ml) 3 times a day. For acute conditions, take 1 tablespoon (15 ml) each hour.
Diluted in tea: As a preventative, take 1 tablespoon (15 ml) in tea 3 times a day. For acute conditions, 1 tablespoon (15 ml) in tea 6 to 10 times a day.

The Best Cold and Flu Tea

2 teaspoons sage
Juice of one lemon (or 1 teaspoon
   lemon balm herb)
Pinch cayenne pepper
1 tablespoon (15 ml) honey

Pour 1 cup boiling water over sage and allow to steep for 10 minutes. Strain out herbs, add remaining ingredients, and drink hot.

Side Effects and Contraindications

External Use: none.

Internal Use: There are three instances where honey can be harmful. 1) Bees sometimes make honey from poisonous plants and these plant poisons can affect people who eat the honey. Though this is very rare it does sometimes occur. Usually honey bought from reliable beekeepers or local sources who know which plants their honeybees use is safe. 2) Occasionally, uncooked honeys can contain botulism spores that can be quite dangerous to children under one year old. The Centers for Disease Control recommends avoiding honey for these young children. Their digestive systems are more fully formed after one year and there are no reports of adverse reactions after that age. You may wish to wait as long as two years to be sure. 3) In rare instances people with allergic reactions to bee stings may have adverse reactions to honey.

Alternatives to Honey

Cell regeneration and antibacterial action: echinacea, aloe.

Wound and burn healing without scarring: aloe, St. John's wort.

Antibacterial action on wounds: goldenseal, usnea, wormwood, sage, garlic, cryptolepsis.

JUNIPER (*Juniperus* spp.)

Family: Cupressaceae.

Part used: Usually berries and needles, but the bark, wood, and root are all active.

Collection: Gather needles, bark, roots, or heartwood at any time. First-year berries, which are green, should be gathered after the first frost, second-year berries, which are bluish-purple, at any time. The berries are ripe when they turn bluish-purple.

Actions: Antibacterial, antimicrobial, antiseptic, antifungal, carminative, anticatarrhal.

Active against: *Staphylococcus aureus, Pseudomonas aeruginosa, Shigella dysenteriae, Streptococcus* spp., *Escherichia coli, Candida albicans, Salmonella* spp.

About Juniper

The evergreens have a traditional use in every culture on Earth for purifying and cleansing: physically, emotionally, and spiritually. They represent incorruptibility and have been used for preventing decay for millennia. They have been used in sweat baths or saunas by nearly every culture throughout time to help prevent or cure illness. Their use by indigenous cultures is pervasive, and scores of scientific studies have supported this historical use. The essential oil of the berries is excreted in the urine and is antibacterial against the antibiotic-resistant bacteria that cause urinary tract infections. *In vitro* studies have shown strong activity against antibiotic-resistant bacteria, especially *Staphylococcus aureus*.

Preparation and Dosage

The berries are used to treat urinary tract infections. The berries or needles are used for upper respiratory infections, *Salmonella*, *E. coli*, *Shigella*. The heartwood, roots, bark, berries, or needles are used for skin infections and infectious dysentery. Essential oil is used for airborne and upper respiratory infections. May be used in food, as tea, wash, tincture, whole, powdered, steam.

Tincture: Berries: 1:5 with 75 percent alcohol, 5 to 30 drops up to 3 times a day.

Tea: 1 teaspoon ground needles steeped in 6 ounces (177 ml) boiling water for 15 minutes, covered. For upper respiratory infections or food poisoning, take as often as desired. For shigella, drink as much tea as can be consumed. As a general preventative and stimulant to the system, drink the tea daily.

Wash: A strong decoction of the herb has been traditionally used in many cultures to sterilize brewing equipment, cooking utensils, surgical instruments, hands,

Source of Vitamin C

One of the often overlooked attributes of the evergreens is their vitamin C content. All animals except the higher primates synthesize their own vitamin C. The new spring growth of the evergreens is lighter in color, less astringent, and decidedly more citrus-tasting than older growth (it has a definite lemon-lime flavor). This new growth has traditionally been used in the human diet in scores of cultures as a source of vitamin C, a vitamin that research has shown contributes significantly to healthy immune functioning (see chapter 4).

counters, etc. The tea is also effective as a wound wash to either prevent or cure infection. Use 1 ounce (25 g) herb per 1 quart (1 l) water, boil 30 minutes, let steep overnight.

Berries: For gastric problems: eat 1 to 5 berries per day for 2 weeks.

Powdered: Add any part of the plant to wound powders, or use alone to prevent or cure infection in wounds.

Food: Berries and new needle growth can be added to many dishes both for flavor and to kill food-borne bacteria. Crumble the berries, or dice new needle growth and cook into food.

Steam: Any part of the plant, but usually the needles or berries. Use in sweat lodge or sauna, or boil 4 ounces (100 g) of needles or crushed berries (fresh is better) in 1 gallon (4 l) water and inhale the steam.

Essential oil: Combine 8 to 10 drops with 1 ounce (30 ml) of water in a nasal spray bottle for sinus and upper respiratory infections. In diffuser for helping prevent and cure upper respiratory infections. Moderate amounts in water for use as steam inhalant or in sweat lodge for upper respiratory infections.

Side Effects and Contraindications

Avoid if you are suffering from acute kidney disease, are pregnant, or have gastric inflammation. High doses or long-term use may irritate kidneys.

Alternatives to Juniper

Any evergreen species, especially pine, fir, cedar, and spruce, in that order. Pine has shown significant antibacterial activity in laboratory study against antibiotic-resistant bacteria, as has fir and, to a lesser extent, spruce. This tends to bear out their long traditional use for healing infectious disease. Dosages for all the evergreens are comparable. The berries of any juniper species may be used similarly.

One relatively new discovery is the power of pine bark in treating disease. Pine bark is higher than any other plant except grapeseed in proanthocyanidin, a powerful antioxidant and potentiator of vitamin C. Free radicals have been implicated in scores of diseases such as cancer, Alzheimer's disease, Parkinson's disease, arthritis, cataracts, heart disease, and stroke. The human immune system uses antioxidants to deactivate and eliminate free radicals from our bodies. This antioxidant from pine bark is one of the strongest known. Furthermore, studies have shown that it powerfully activates the vitamin C in pine needles, a potent historical treatment for scurvy, a vitamin C deficiency disease. There is some evidence that the barks of other evergreen species also possess this same powerful antioxidant activity.

LICORICE *(Glycyrrhiza glabra)*

Family: Leguminosae.
Part used: The root.
Collection: Usually commercially grown, not available wild in North America. Usually picked in early spring or fall when the leaves begin to die back.
Actions: Antioxidant, antidiuretic, smooth muscle relaxant, antispasmodic, immunostimulant (stimulates interferon production, enhances antibody formation, stimulates phagocytosis, antistressor, adrenal tonic, thymus stimulant), antiulcer, anti-inflammatory, tumor inhibitor, free radical inhibitor, antihepatoxic, antimalarial, protects from effects of radiation exposure, gentle laxative, expectorant, demulcent, immunomodulator, antihyperglycemic, reduces gastric secretions, stimulates pancreatic secretions.
Active against: Malaria, tuberculosis, *Bacillus subtilis, Staphylococcus aureus, Streptococcus sobrinus, S. mutans, Salmonella typhimurium, Escherichia coli, Candida albicans, Vibrio cholera, Trichophyton mentagrophytes, T. rubrum, Toxocara canis.*

About Licorice

Licorice, made famous by the rubberoid candy of the same name (which these days may contain *no* licorice because of overdose problems), is a rather remarkable herb. Though I don't primarily think of licorice as an antibacterial herb, the list of organisms against which it is specific is comprehensive and well documented. Generally, it is an immune system stimulant that has impressive antibacterial activity and potentiates the action of other herbs. One distinct advantage of licorice is its sweetness. Fifty times sweeter than sugar, licorice, when used in herbal combinations, helps brighten the awful taste of some herbal formulations, making them more palatable for children and for adults with a strong inner child. (Stoics usually like their herbal preparations bitter.)

Unlike many herbs, licorice has a long history of clinical human trials; its side effects and strengths are well documented. It is specific for upper respiratory infections, coughs, colds, and ulcerations anywhere in the gastrointestinal tract, especially the stomach. It is highly useful for helping repair damaged adrenals, and this helps restore overall system health and vitality. There is good evidence that it stimulates the thymus gland, one of the most important organs in the immune system, in that extremely large doses in rats begin to destroy that organ and it decreases substantially in weight. Scientific studies have shown that licorice increases the generation and activity of white blood cells, stimulates interferon production in the body, and enhances antibody formation. Several trials have shown that it also possesses a distinct immunomodulator activity. That is, if the immune system is overactive, licorice calms it down; if underactive, it pumps its up.

Licorice has shown distinct antifatigue and antistress activity, and *in vivo* studies have shown strong activity against cancerous tumors and some protection from the effects of radiation. Perhaps it is best known for its estrogenic effects, which make it a useful herb for menopause, and its antiulcer activity, making it an herb of choice for both stomach and duodenal ulceration. Because it stimulates expectoration and is powerfully healing for mucous membrane systems, it has a long history of use for upper respiratory infections.

The best way to use licorice is in combination with other herbs, especially for bacteria for which it is specific. Used in proper doses in moderation, licorice is one of the most powerful members of the herbal family. It may be used for restoring immune function or in active disease conditions. It is especially useful for any mucous membrane infection, cancer, radiation treatment, general fatigue, or immune suppression.

Go for Organic

Most of the licorice in commerce comes from Eastern Europe, which possesses some of the highest levels of soil and air pollution in the world. It makes no sense to buy potentially contaminated herbs that have broad-spectrum immune and liver actions. Organically grown licorice is much better. If you buy both and compare them, you will find a significant difference in quality.

Because of the many potential side effects from overuse or large doses, caution should be exercised in its use.

Preparation and Dosage

Used as tea, in capsules, as tincture.

Tincture: Dried root, 1:5 with 50 percent alcohol, 30 to 60 drops up to 3 times a day.

Tea: ½ to 1 teaspoon (2 to 5 ml) of powdered root in 8 ounces (237 ml) water, simmer 15 minutes, strain. Drink up to 3 cups a day.

Capsules: 2 to 8 double-ought capsules per day.

Side Effects and Contraindications

Many. Because of licorice's many strengths, a lot of people overuse it, with sometimes serious side effects. Overdoses or long use of large doses can cause severe potassium depletion (hypokalemia), hypertension, decrease in plasma renin and aldosterone levels, edema, and at very large doses decreased body and thymus weight and blood cell counts. Because of the strong estrogenic activity of licorice, it will also cause breast growth in men, especially when combined with other estrogenic herbs. Luckily, all these conditions tend to abate within 2 to 4 weeks after licorice intake ceases. Caution should be used, however, in length and strength of dosages. Contraindicated in hypertension, hypokalemia, pregnancy, and hypernatremia, and in persons taking estrogen therapy or corticosteroids. Daniel Mowrey, in his *Herbal Tonic Therapies* (Wings Books, 1993), suggests that the side effects from licorice are all from licorice extracts and none are from use of the whole plant (i.e., the ground root) taken in capsules. The citations I have found for side effects are generally for licorice candy or extracts. Mowrey comments that this propensity of licorice to cause side effects when extracts are used supports the use of the plant itself, which often contains other compounds that ameliorate the side effects of extracted constituents.

Alternatives to Licorice

The American species, found wild throughout North America, though not sweet can be reliably substituted.

SAGE *(Salvia officinalis)*

Family: Labiateae.
Part used: The leaves.
Collection: This is the culinary sage of commerce. The plant is indigenous to southern Europe but is now naturalized throughout the world. Harvest the leaves just before flowering in early summer. Dry in the shade.
Actions: Antiseptic, antibacterial, astringent, tonic, expectorant, diaphoretic.
Active against: *Streptococcus pneumoniae, Staphylococcus aureus, Haemophilus influenzae, Pseudomonas aeruginosa, Escherichia coli, Candida albicans, Klebsiella pneumoniae, Salmonella* spp. The essential oil is a broad-spectrum antibiotic.

About Sage

Especially good for dysentery, throat and upper respiratory infections, or any infection with excess secretions; used externally for infected wounds. Though not as strong as some other herbs, the sages have been used for at least two millennia in all cultures where they grow for persistent bacterial infections within and without the body. Laboratory studies have verified their long-standing antibacterial activity. Their moderate yet consistent antibacterial activity and good taste make them especially useful because of their traditional use in food. Furthermore, their good taste and reliable action make them especially suited for children.

Preparation and Dosage

May be used as tea, tincture, inhalant, smoke, powder, essential oil, and food additive.
Tea: 2 teaspoons leaf in 8 ounces (237 ml) water, steep 15 minutes. Gargle and then drink for active throat infections and fevers 3 to 6 times a day. *For tonic use:* steep 4 ounces (113 g) in 1 quart (1 l) water overnight and drink cold throughout the next day, up to 7 days.
Tincture: Fresh herb 1:2 with 95 percent alcohol; dry herb 1:5 with 50 percent alcohol. *For prevention:* 10 to 30 drops up to 3 times a day. In acute conditions: 30 to 60 drops up to 6 times a day.

Inhalant: 4 ounces (113 g) herb in 1 gallon (4 l) of water, bring to a boil, inhale steam.

Smoke: Place herb or tea on stones in sweat lodge or sauna.

Powder: On all external infected wounds.

Essential oil: In diffuser or a few drops in 1 ounce (30 ml) water in inhaler as nasal spray. Using it in a diffuser helps prevent and cure infection and lightens the spirits.

Food/Cooking: To combat food pathogens, use liberally in daily diet.

Side Effects and Contraindications

Sage will decrease or even stop lactation in a nursing mother. Not suggested in large quantities during pregnancy.

Sage Advantage

Note: Most salvias can be used in much the same way. Generally, white sage is stronger than its culinary cousin, but overall the sages are not as strong as the wormwoods, with which they are often confused. Though they have similar antibacterial and antiseptic action, the wormwoods are bitter and *increase* secretions in the body. The sages are tasty and *decrease* secretions.

Alternatives to Sage

The artemisias (though not in food — they are exceptionally bitter). In food, thyme and rosemary are alternatives.

USNEA (*Usnea* spp.)

Family: Parmeliaceae.

Part used: Whole lichen.

Collection: Usnea is an extremely prolific though slow-growing, long-lived, gray-green to yellow-green lichen growing on trees throughout the world. The whole lichen may be harvested at any time.

Actions: Antibacterial, antifungal, immune stimulant.

Active against: Tuberculosis, *Pneumonococcus* spp., *Staphlycoccus aureus*, enterococcus, *Streptococcus* spp., *Trichomonas*, *Candida* spp., various fungal strains. Generally active against gram-positive bacteria. Though it is supposedly not effective against gram-negative bacteria, one *in vitro* study found usnea to be specific against *Salmonella typhimurium*, and at least one journal reports effectiveness against *Escherichia coli*.

About Usnea

Commonly called old man's beard, a name derived from its appearance, usnea is a lichen that grows on living and dead trees throughout the world. It is quite common in North America, and this wide availability and its strong antibacterial properties make it a significant herb in treating resistant bacteria.

Usnea ranges in size from a small tuft to large hanging strands resembling hair. It may be gray-green in the smaller species and mild yellow-green in the larger hanging strands. The herb is a symbiote composed of two plants intertwined. The inner plant is a thin white thread, which when wet stretches like a rubber band. The outer plant gives the herb its color and grows around the inner rubber-band–like plant. The distinctive method of identifying usnea is wetting it and stretching it to see whether it is springy and, when it snaps apart, looking for the distinctive white thread of the inner plant. This inner band is strongly immune stimulating, and the outer plant sheath possesses strong antibiotic properties.

While generally inactive against gram-negative bacteria, usnea has strong antibiotic activity against gram-positive bacteria. At dilutions of 1:20,000 to 1:50,000, usnea was found to completely inhibit the growth of tuberculosis, and in dilutions of 1:20,000, it completely inhibited the growth of *Staphylococcus, Streptococcus,* and *Pneumonococcus* organisms. In fact, it has shown activity more effective against some bacterial strains than penicillin. In studies carried out in the early part of this century, over 52 different species of lichen besides usnea were shown to inhibit bacterial growth. Compounds in the lichens that inhibit bacteria are usnic acid, protolichesterinic acid, some orcinol derivatives, and several (as usual) unidentified substances. Of those, the strongest is usnic acid, present in all usnea species.

Usnea has been traditionally used throughout the world for skin infections, abscesses, upper respiratory and lung infections, vaginal infections, and fungal infections. The lichen, soaked in garlic juice or a strong garlic decoction, was one traditional method of treating large gaping wounds in the body.

Preparation and Dosage

May be used externally as a tincture, wash, or powder. May be used internally as a tea, tincture, spray, or douche.

External bacterial or fungal infections: As a powder liberally sprinkled on site of infection as frequently as needed, except for impetigo (staphylococcal or streptococcal infection of the skin): use the tinture full strength or 50 percent dilute tinture applied directly on site of infection with cotton swab.

> ### Getting the Most from Usnea
>
> Usnea is only partially water soluble. To make the strongest tea or decoction, grind the herb first, then add enough alcohol to wet the herb, let it sit covered for 30 minutes, add hot water, and let steep.

<u>Internal Uses:</u>

Tincture: 1:5 with 50 percent alcohol. (*Note:* usnea is not easily soluble in alcohol unless it is mechanically ground first. The outer, green sheath will powder; the inner cord will remain unpowdered and appear much like a ball of white hair. Both will give up their constituents to an alcohol/water combination). As a preventative or for immune stimulation: 30 to 60 drops up to 4 times a day. For acute bacterial infections, including tuberculosis: 1 teaspoon (5 ml) up to 6 times a day.

Tea: For disease prevention or immune stimulation: 1 teaspoon (5 ml) herb in 6 ounces (177 ml) hot water, steep 20 minutes; 2 to 6 ounces (59 to 177 ml) up to 3 times a day. In acute conditions: up to 1 quart (1 l) a day.

Nasal spray: 10 drops in water in nasal sprayer; use as needed for colds and flu.

Douche for vaginal infections: ½ ounce (15 ml) tinture in 1 pint (475 ml) water. Douche 2 times a day, upon rising and before retiring, for 3 days.

Side Effects and Contraindications

Usnea tincture is often irritating to the mucous membranes of the mouth and throat; it should be diluted in a glass of water (or any suitable liquid) before consumption.

Though animal testing has shown that excessively large amounts of usnic acid, one of the components of usnea, is toxic to animals, no toxicity has been noted in human use. Usnea also readily absorbs heavy metals in potentially toxic amounts. This is particularly problematic in far northern latitudes. Generally, the amount of usnea taken internally will not contain sufficient amounts of heavy metals to present a problem. In order to avoid such problems, harvest usnea at least 300 feet from roads, factories, and polluted areas.

Alternatives to Usnea

Any usnea species, Iceland moss *(Cetraria islandica)* for mucous membrane systems, garlic.

WORMWOOD *(Artemisia absinthium)*

Family: Compositae.
Part used: The entire plant.
Collection: Wormwood grows throughout the world. The above-ground plant is most often used for medicine, and it may be harvested at any time. The root, a powerful medicine in its own right, is rarely used as medicine; it too may be harvested at any time.
Actions: *Herb:* Antibacterial, antimalarial, antifungal, immunomodulator, anthelmintic, anti-inflammatory, diaphoretic, antihepatoxic, euphoriant, antiamoebic, antipyretic, gastric stimulant, choleretic, bitter tonic, smooth muscle relaxant. *Root:* antibacterial, immunostimulant, diaphoretic, antipyretic.
Active against: Malaria, *Staphlycoccus aureus*, *Naegleria floweri*, *Pseudomonas aeruginosa*, *Candida albicans*, *Klebsiella pneumoniae*, intestinal worms, any internal amebic organisms. The essential oil is effective against most microbes.

About Wormwood

Though the root is rarely used for medicine, it is extremely powerful, especially for hot, sore infections of the throat and lungs. It numbs pain from infection in the throat and bronchial tubes and is exceptionally cooling to the throat and lungs. It is also highly antibacterial, being exceptionally effective topically. The leaf or above-ground plant is generally used for malaria, for intestinal worms, as a liver and digestive tonic, and for colds and flu. Water infusions of the leaf have been shown to produce 89 percent inhibition of malaria at 1 part in 35. Regular use as a tea *as a preventative* was found to prevent acetaminophen-induced liver disease in mice and rats. Some herbalists do not recommend the use of this herb because of its thujone content. However, it is one of the most powerful herbs for the treatment of antibiotic-resistant disease available. Millennia of traditional use support its continued place in the herbal dispensatory.

Inevitably, medical researchers have insisted on isolating a chemical component of wormwood, called artemesinin, for use in treating malaria. Artemesinin has been further processed into a specific drug, artemether. Clinical trials have shown that artemether is as effective as quinine in treating both resistant and nonresistant strains of malaria; trials in Gambia and Vietnam showed similar results. In the Vietnamese study, malarial symptoms cleared in 30 hours with artemether, 33 hours with quinine. Parasite clearance was markedly shorter with artemether in all trials; in the Vietnamese study it was 48 hours, versus 60 hours with quinine. However, patients given artemether experienced several unpleasant side effects from the drug (as is often the case with pharmaceuticals). As with all searches for "active constituents" there is some question about its necessity.

Using Artemisia Species

Note: All artemisia species may be used similarly. The mildest is mugwort, *Artemisia vulgaris;* the two most powerful are wormwood and sweet Annie, *Artemisia annua.* The latter is used extensively throughout Asia for malaria with great success. (For malaria: 25 to 40 milligrams of leafy herb per kilogram [3 pounds] of body weight 3 times a day before meals for 7 days.) Like cryptolepsis, it was a traditional fever and malarial herb that has been rediscovered for the treatment of antibiotic-resistant malaria. Wormwood may be used likewise, and generally it is a bit easier to find. Recent research on one constituent of the artemisias, artemesinin, has shown reliable immunomodulation activity, making the constituent and the herb useful in treating autoimmune disorders.

Taiwanese researchers have found the whole herb to be as effective with fewer side effects than the isolated component. Furthermore, extracts of *Artemisia annua* that contained *no* artemesinin were just as effective an antimalarial (though at twice the dosage for artemesinin).

Preparation and Dosage

The above-ground plant may be used as tea, tincture, capsules, smoke, or essential oil, or in whole form.

Tea: Hot tea for antipyretic and diaphoretic effects: 8 ounces (236 ml) of boiling water per 1 or 2 ounces (25 or 50 g) of herb, steeped for 15 minutes, taken as needed for fevers, colds, flu. Cold tea for use as a tonic: 4 ounces (113 g) of herb in 1 quart (1 l) hot water, steep overnight, strain, drink throughout the day up to 7 days.

Tincture: Fresh plant 1:2 with 95 percent alcohol, dried plant 1:5 with 50 percent alcohol, 10 to 30 drops up to 6 times a day.

Capsules: 1 to 5 double-ought capsules up to 4 times a day.

Smoke: In sweat lodge or sauna, or as rolled cigarettes.

Root: As tincture or in whole form.

Tincture of dried root: 1:5 with 60 percent alcohol, use 10 to 30 drops up to 4 times a day for active infections.

Whole root: Cut small pieces of root (¼ inch [6¼ mm] long) and eat fresh as often as desired for upper respiratory infections. *Note:* the above-ground plant is extremely bitter; the root is not.

Essential oil: Extremely useful in the home when used in a diffuser for all airborne bacteria. It is exceptionally toxic if used internally.

Side Effects and Contraindications

Avoid large doses during pregnancy. Concentrated infusions have caused abortion in rats, though weak teas are considered safe. The essential oil is *never* appropriate to take internally: small doses cause acute renal insufficiency and death. Extensive overuse of the herb over years may result in central nervous system damage from the high levels of thujone (a narcotic poison) in the plant.

Caution: Some herbalists feel that the presence of thujone, and the possible nervous system damage from it, is too dangerous to risk using wormwood at all. Many other herbalists have used the herb for many years with no sign of adverse reactions. Use in folk practice throughout the world is pervasive. It should be recognized, however, that wormwood is a strong herb and should be used with respect and attentiveness of mind.

Alternatives to Wormwood

Any artemisia species, cryptolepsis. Any artemisia can be substituted for another; however, *Artemisia vulgaris,* mugwort, is the least strong of the artemisias and will probably prove an ineffective choice for treatment of malaria. Dosage will vary depending on species.

HERBAL TREATMENTS FOR 12 COMMON ANTIBIOTIC-RESISTANT MICROBES

MICROBE/ DISEASES CAUSED	EFFECTIVE HERBAL TREATMENTS
Enterococcus Surgical infections, Blood poisoning	**For surgical wounds:** external applications of usnea, echinacea, garlic, grapefruit seed extract, eucalyptus, honey, witch hazel *(Hamamelis virginiana)* **For blood poisoning:** echinacea (massive doses); garlic (massive doses); usnea (massive doses)
Haemophilus influenzae Meningitis, Ear infections, Pneumonia, Sinusitis	Coltsfoot *(Tussilago farfara* is specific for this bacterium), garlic, goldenseal, sage, oak bark, boneset, grapefruit seed extract (and for pneumonia, essential oils of thyme or oregano)
Mycobacterium tuberculosis Tuberculosis	Garlic, usnea, grapefruit seed extract, boneset, goldenseal, red clover *(Trifolium pratense)*, shizandra *(Schisandra chinensis)*, elecampane *(Inula helenium)*
Neisseria gonorrhoeae Gonorrhea	Garlic, acacia, large spotted spurge *(Euphorbia hypericifolia)*, *Cassia abbreviata*
Plasmodium falciparum Malaria	Cryptolepsis, artemisia, *Uvaria* spp., *Brucea javanica,* garlic vine *(Mansoa standleyi)*
Pseudomonas aeruginosa Pneumonia, Urinary tract infections, Bacteremia	**For pneumonia:** aloe, eucalyptus, juniper, garlic, *Cassia* spp., grapefruit seed extract, essential oils of thyme or oregano. Large spotted spurge *(Euphorbia hypericifolia),* spotted spurge *(E. maculata), Euphorbia lathyris.* **For urinary tract infections:** juniper, uva ursi *(Arctostaphylos uva-ursi),* eucalyptus, goldenseal, cranberry. *Cassia Fistula* and five other Cassia species have been found effective in vitro against Pseudomonas aeruginosa. *C. Fistula* is excreted in the urine and thus should be good for UTI. **For bacteremia:** echinacea, massive doses; garlic, massive doses; boneset, massive doses
Shigella dysenteriae Severe diarrhea	Goldenseal, garlic, grapefruit seed extract, *Terminalia* spp., cryptolepsis, sage, oak

chart continued on page 64

HERBAL TREATMENTS FOR 12 COMMON ANTIBIOTIC-RESISTANT MICROBES

MICROBE/ DISEASES CAUSED	EFFECTIVE HERBAL TREATMENTS
Staphylococcus aureus Pneumonia, Surgical infections, Bacteremia	**For pneumonia:** usnea, garlic, goldenseal, cryptolepsis, eucalyptus, boneset, wormwood, *Terminalia* spp., juniper, *Withania* spp., *Populus* spp., grapefruit seed extract, essential oils of thyme or oregano **For surgical/skin infections:** usnea, garlic, cryptolepsis, eucalyptus, wormwood, sage, honey, St. John's wort *(Hypericum perforatum)*, *Withania* spp., juniper, *Cassia* spp., *Terminalia* spp., grapefruit seed extract **For bacteremia:** echinacea, massive doses; garlic, massive doses; usnea, massive doses; boneset, massive doses
Streptococcus pneumoniae Meningitis, Pneumonia	Garlic, usnea, echinacea (for strep throat), eucalyptus, ginger, sage, rosemary *(Rosmarinus officinalis)*, boneset, grapefruit seed extract, lavender *(Lavandula officinalis)*
Klebsiella pneumoniae Pneumonia, Urinary tract and surgical wound infections, Bacteremia	**For urinary tract infections:** eucalyptus, juniper, uva ursi, goldenseal **For pneumonia:** ginger, goldenseal, grapefruit seed extract, sage, wormwood, boneset, essential oils of thyme or oregano, pleurisy root *(Asclepias tuberusa)* **For surgical wound infections:** eucalyptus, ginger, goldenseal, sage, wormwood **For bacteremia:** echinacea, massive doses; garlic, massive doses
Escherichia coli Virulent strains of food poisoning, Severe bloody diarrhea	Goldenseal, garlic, eucalyptus, cryptolepsis, juniper, acacia, sage, ginger, grapefruit seed extract
Salmonella **spp.** Food poisoning, Severe diarrhea	Garlic, eucalyptus, wormwood, juniper, goldenseal, sage, ginger, acacia, grapefruit seed extract, *Terminalia* spp., *Punica* spp.

ANTIBACTERIAL HERBS
FOR FOOD-BORNE PATHOGENS

As noted in the first chapter, the contamination of our food supply with resistant bacteria is becoming a serious problem, and it is likely to worsen as population increases. It turns out, however, that herbs have been used in our foods for millennia for protecting us from infectious and pathogenic disease.

A group of researchers at Cornell University found in an examination of traditional food preparations that as local climate temperature increases the number of spices used in food also increases. That is, in hot climates a lot of spices are used; in cold climates, almost none (the cold weather itself protects food supplies). In examining the spices most commonly used, they found that they all possessed powerful antimicrobial activity. The most powerful of the herbs tested were garlic, onion, allspice, and oregano, which killed 100 percent of the food-borne bacteria for which the researchers tested. The study, not surprisingly, found that many spices are synergists and when combined exhibit antibacterial action much stronger than they do alone. These multiple spice combinations produce the most powerful antimicrobial effects when salt and lemon or lime juice is also added during cooking.

Powerful Spice Blends

Some of the most powerful traditional blends of spices are chili powder (capsicums, onion, paprika, garlic, cumin, oregano), five-spice powder (white or black pepper, cinnamon, anise, fennel, cloves), salsa (capsicums, onion, garlic, tomatoes, lime), and curry powder (tumeric [a potent antibacterial antifungal, antiparasitic, and antiviral herb], curry leaves [a potent antiamebic, antimalarial, and antidiarrheal herb], cumin, cardamom, ginger, mustard, coriander).

Some of the spices, though only killing about 25 percent of the number of bacteria types tested, were exceptionally strong against one or two bacteria alone. Among them are rosemary, thyme, marjoram, sage, and lemon or lime juice. All the spices listed in the box on page 66 are noted in the University Of Chicago NAPRALERT database, one of the most extensive herbal data bases in the world, as showing antibacterial activity in *in vitro, in vivo,* or human trials.

Oddly, even though the researchers note that juniper is used as a spice in every region in which it grows (making it one of the top five cooking spices in the world), they did not search the literature for its antimicrobial activity. A correlation with its antimicrobial activity would place it in the top six or seven spices for antipathogenic activity.

EFFECTIVENESS OF ANTIBACTERIAL SPICES

Note: The spices are listed in descending order of strength, according to findings of Cornell University research study.

Kill 100 percent of bacteria: garlic, onions, allspice, oregano

Kill 90 to 75 percent of bacteria: thyme, cinnamon, tarragon, cumin, cloves, lemongrass, bay leaf, capsicums, rosemary, marjoram, mustard

Kill 72 to 50 percent of bacteria: caraway, mint, sage, fennel, coriander, dill, nutmeg, basil, parsley

Kill 48 to 25 percent of bacteria: cardamom, pepper, ginger, anise seed, celery seed, lemon or lime juice

3

THE FIRST LINE OF DEFENSE: STRENGTHENING THE IMMUNE SYSTEM

Generally, no matter how virulent a disease — and this includes fearsome diseases like that caused by the Ebola virus — many people remain healthy in spite of being exposed. In fact, medical studies have consistently shown the presence of virulent bacteria in many peoples' systems though they themselves never become ill. Unfortunately, few studies have been conducted on why these people do not get ill; most of the focus has been on "fighting" the disease. But those people who do not get ill all have something in common that their ill neighbors do not: their immune systems successfully keep an infection from taking over their bodies. Our immune systems are, in fact, our first line of defense. The job of the immune system is to protect us from disease and, if disease occurs, to cure it. A healthy immune system, then, is the most important thing we can possess to help us remain healthy.

> The man is not sick because he has an illness; he has an illness because he is sick.
>
> *CHINESE PROVERB*

SUPPORTING THE ELEMENTS OF THE IMMUNE SYSTEM

Some of the specific components of our immune system are the thymus, spleen, lymph system, lymph nodes, tonsils, liver, appendix (basically a large lymph node), and bone marrow. The thymus coordinates immune activity. The spleen processes worn-out red blood cells and platelets and provides a location to engulf and destroy invading bacteria. The liver cleans toxins from the blood and produces most of the body's lymph, the liquid that flows in the lymph system, basically the body's sewer system. This system runs parallel to the blood vessels; it stores, filters, and circulates waste, especially dead bacteria and the massive numbers of white blood cells produced during active infections. Lymph nodes are large intersections of lymph channels, and they store or warehouse the waste products being processed through the lymph system. When the lymph nodes are processing a lot of waste they tend to swell, clog up, and become painful to the touch, and processing of waste slows down. Keeping the nodes clear helps the body process infections much quicker. The lymph nodes (as does the thymus gland) also produce unique white blood cells called lymphocytes that are potent elements of our immune system.

The bone marrow and to some extent the thymus manufacture other types of white blood cells to fight infections. Two of the most important are phagocytes and neutrophils. Phagocytes exist in three forms: monocytes, macrophages, and granulocytes. As macrophages they rove the body looking for foreign bodies, engulf invading bacteria, and help clean up residues of white blood cells and bacteria during and after infections. They also alert the neutrophils, which attack and destroy bacteria and viruses, to the presence of disease organisms.

All the differing parts of this whole immune complex can be supported and kept healthy. By doing so we help prevent inroads in our systems from antibiotic-resistant bacteria.

Revitalizing Strategies

Over the past three decades there has been a great deal of exploration of just what is involved in creating and maintaining overall health and vitality. This includes things that can be done to restore and revitalize a suppressed or damaged immune system or keep an already healthy immune system functioning well. Roughly, these measures fall into three categories: herbs, foods and vitamins, and lifestyle choices.

A basic truism of antibiotic treatment is that it just will not work under most circumstances unless the body can mount its own attack against invading bacteria.

MARC LAPPÉ, PH.D.

HERBS FOR THE IMMUNE SYSTEM

Several herbs stand out when it comes to strengthening, rehabilitating, or enhancing the immune system. All of them can be used over the long term; few have any side effects. Though some of them are active against specific disease organisms, their strength lies in enhancing various aspects of the immune system, offering protective activity against toxins or disease for specific organs in the body, antitumor activity, and/or tonifying and restoring a debilitated body or immune system. Many of these herbs are also considered antistressors. They seem to protect the body from the effects of stress — and stress, it has been shown, will actually impair immune effectiveness over time.

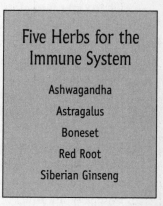

Five Herbs for the Immune System

Ashwagandha

Astragalus

Boneset

Red Root

Siberian Ginseng

ASHWAGANDHA *(Withania somnifera)*

Family: Solanaceae.

Part used: The root is used in Western practice; all parts of the plant are used in the rest of the world.

Collection: The plant is little grown (or known) in this country but common in India, Sudan, Pakistan, Iraq, Saudi Arabia, and Rwanda. The root is usually harvested in the fall; the leaves, at any time; the seeds, in season.

Actions: Root: immune tonic, stress-protective, antibacterial, diuretic, antipyretic, astringent, nerve sedative, alterative.

Leaves and stem: antipyretic, febrifuge, bitter, diuretic, antibacterial, antimicrobial, astringent, nerve sedative.

Seeds: hypnotic, diuretic, coagulant.

Fruit (of related species): immune tonic, antibacterial, alterative.

Active against: *Staphylococcus aureus, Pseudomonas aeruginosa, Salmonella* spp.

About Ashwagandha

Ashwagandha has a reputation as a strong and sure immune tonic and stress protector, rivaling ginseng in the few clinical trials conducted. It has a millennia-long tradition of use in Northern Africa, India, and portions of Asia. One of its strengths is its sure and reliable action as a nerve sedative. For people who are highly stressed, the herb gently lowers stress levels in the body, protects the body from stress-related disease, and brings the immune system up to optimum levels of activity. As with most immune tonics (as opposed to immune stimulants like echinacea), the herb works best over time. Like Siberian ginseng, it will take 6 weeks to 6 months to get a good sense whether the herb will work for you.

Two other *Withania* species are used in much the same manner: *W. obtusifolia* and *W. coagulans*. *W. obtusifolia* has a long history of use in the Sudan, and *W. coagulans* (especially the fruit) has long been used in Pakistan and India. *W. coagulans* is so termed because it is a powerful coagulating agent and is used in place of rennet by Indians to make cheese.

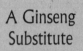

A Ginseng Substitute

Similar in its effects to ginseng, ashwagandha is much cheaper, not yet being an "herb-of-the-day" in the West.

Preparation and Dosage

Ashwagandha is available almost exclusively through larger health food stores. Prepare powdered root as single or double-ought capsules; taken 1 to 6 per day.

Side Effects and Contraindications

Used in India as an abortifacient. Not suggested for use during pregnancy. The root and leaves are considered narcotic, as are many members of the *Solanaceae* family; the seeds are considered a hypnotic narcotic. Caution is suggested in ingesting large doses. However, the record of folk use indicates that the narcotic effects of the herb are not nearly as strong as those of its cousin henbane (*Hyoscyamus niger*) and are slightly stronger than those of its relative dulcamara (*Solanum dulcamara*). The plant is fairly high in nicotine, so those trying to quit smoking may find that this herb makes that task more difficult.

Alternatives to Ashwangandha

Siberian ginseng, astragalus, ginseng (for those over 40), and two other *Withania* species: *W. coagulans* and *W. obtusifolia*.

ASTRAGALUS *(Astragalus membranaceus)*

Family: Leguminosae.
Part used: The plant is a perennial with a long fibrous root stock. The root is used for medicine.
Collection: The plant grows in Asia and is primarily harvested in China, having been used in Chinese medicine for millennia. The root is thinly sliced and dried, and it most closely resembles a yellow tongue depressor.
Actions: Immune enhancer, stimulant, and restorative; antiviral; adaptogen; tonic; diuretic; enhances function in lungs, spleen, and digestion.
Active against: *Staphylococcus aureus*, *Salmonella* spp., *Proteus mirabilis*.

About Astragalus

Astragalus has been found to be exceptionally effective for the immune system. Clinical studies have shown that astragalus both protects the human heart from Coxsackie b 2 virus and helps repair damage in previously infected people. Other studies have shown that astragalus enhances the body's own natural killer cell activity. As an antitumor agent, astragalus prevented cancer metastasis in 80 percent of mice tested. Still other studies have shown that astragalus stimulates T-cell activity and restores immune function in cancer patients with impaired immune function. The action of astragalus is comprehensive. Robyn Landis and K. P. Khalsa note that "astragalus stimulates phagocytosis (invader-engulfing activity), increasing the total number of cells and the aggressiveness of their activity. Increased macrophage activity has been measured as lasting up to seventy-two hours. It increases the number of stem cells (the 'generic' cells that can become any type needed) in the marrow and lymph tissue, stimulates their maturation into active immune cells, increases spleen activity, increases releases of antibodies, and boosts the production of hormonal messenger molecules that signal for virus destruction." And as Rob McCaleb noted in *HerbalGram* 21 (summer 1988) researchers at the University of Texas Medical Center found that astragalus was able to completely restore the function of cancer patients' compromised immune cells. Finally, research has also shown that astragalus protects the liver from a variety of liver toxins, such as carbon tetrachloride and the anticancer compound stilbenemide. The liver is an important organ in the body's immune support system.

A good way to use astragalus for medicine is to make it into a soup stock or to cook rice in a strong astragalus infusion or tea. Astragalus is quite tasty and has been used this way throughout the world for many thousands of years. The sliced root should be removed after cooking and discarded, as it is too fibrous to eat.

Preparation and Dosage

Astragalus may be taken as tea, in capsules, as tincture, or in food.

Tea: 2 to 3 ounces (50 to 75 g) of herb to a pot of tea; drink throughout the day.

Capsules: Grind herb to powder and encapsulate; take 3 capsules 3 times a day as immune tonic.

Tincture: 1:5 with 60 percent alcohol, 30 to 60 drops up to 4 times a day.

Food: Two of the best ways to use astragalus as food are as a broth base for soups and as a rice (see recipe box).

Side Effects and Contraindications

No toxicity has ever been shown from the ingestion of astragalus. And the Chinese report consistent use for millennia in the treatment of colds and flu and suppressed immune function. This is certainly one of the top herbs to use to restore a depressed or damaged immune system.

Alterantives to Astragalus

Ashwagandha, Siberian ginseng, shiitake mushroom.

Purchasing Astragalus

Astragalus can be quite expensive when purchased from herbal suppliers or health food stores. The same product can be purchased from most Chinese or Asian markets, sometimes for as little as one-tenth the price charged by herbal marketers.

Astragalus Broth

Robyn Landis's and K.P. Khalsa's recipe in Herbal Defense *was the original inspiration for this powerful recipe.*

> 3 cups (750 ml) water or vegetable broth
> ½ cup (or to taste) vegebroth powder*
> (or vegetable soup stock, if desired)
> 6 slices dried astragalus root
> 3 tablespoons dried garlic powder
> or 10 cloves peeled fresh garlic

Place all ingredients in pot and simmer for two to three hours, covered.

To Use: If you feel you are getting sick make and consume the entire recipe. As a preventative take a cup or two during the week. If you use fresh garlic, eat it after the broth is done or as the broth is consumed.

Available from Trinity Herb — see Resources

Immune-Enhancing Rice

> 8 slices dried astragalus root
> 4 cups (1 l) water
> 2 cups brown rice

Add astragalus to water, bring to boil, and simmer for 2 hours, covered. Remove from heat and let stand overnight. Remove astragalus, add water to bring back up to 4 cups (1 l), add rice, and bring to a boil. Reduce heat and simmer until done, approximately 1 hour. Use this rice as you would any rice, as a base for meals throughout the week.

❦BONESET *(Eupatorium perfoliatum)*

Family: Compositae.
Part used: Above-ground plant.
Collection: If allowed to dry, the flowering plant will usually go to seed. It should be collected when it is in flower (August or September) if being tinctured fresh. Otherwise it should be picked just before flowering, hung upside down in a shaded place, and allowed to thoroughly air-dry.
Actions: Immunostimulant (increases phagocytosis to four times that of echinacea), diaphoretic, febrifuge, mucous membrane tonic, smooth muscle relaxant, anti-inflammatory, cytotoxic, mild emetic, peripheral circulatory stimulant, gastric bitter.
Active against: Although many of the *Eupatoriums* have been found active against *Staphlycoccus aureus* and *Pseudomonas aeruginosa*, boneset has not. Traditionally used for dengue fever, malaria, pneumonia, colds, and flu, it has not, to my knowledge, been tested against malaria or dengue fever organisms. Empirically, its strength seems to be for pain relief and as an immunostimulant, a tonic for the mucous membrane systems, and a febrifuge.

About Boneset

To lay the matter straight: There is endless discussion and pontification about how boneset got its name. One school has it that the common name for dengue fever, breakbone fever, was the genesis. Another says that flus and colds were historically called "breakbone fever" in the early colonies and thus gave boneset its name. Still another school insists that the traditional use of boneset by indigenous peoples for healing broken bones (they really did) gave it its name. They are all somewhat correct.

In actuality, boneset has two ancient common names: boneset and ague weed. Ague is an old term for any disease marked by intermittent fever, chills, and pain in the joints and bones. Boneset has a marked ability to allay those conditions, especially bone pain — it settles pain in the bones. Pain in the bones accompanying any ague-like condition is in fact the specific indication for the use of boneset. Dengue fever, a virus transmitted by a mosquito (one of the "new" old epidemics now making inroads from Mexico into the southern United States), is in fact attended by intense pain in the joints and bones, head, eyes, and muscles.

Additionally, there are chills and fever, sore throat, catarrh, and cutaneous eruption. The name boneset attained popularity about 1800 from a particularly virulent flu that swept the East Coast and was attended by intense bone pain. The herbalist Matthew Wood found a specific reference from the early nineteenth-century physician C. J. Hemple, who noted that *Eupatorium perfoliatum* "so singally relieved the disease . . . that it was familiarly called bone-set." Part of the reason why the name boneset might have been adopted in that region at that time is that the Native Americans who used boneset for broken bones were northeastern Indians, and the severe, painful, bone flus that swept the country in 1800 also were confined to the northeast.

The plant, indigenous to North America, was extensively used by native peoples for hundreds if not thousands of years specifically for intermittent fevers and chills, with pain in the bones, weakness, and debility. Interestingly, all *Eupatorium* species are used alike throughout the world. Other species, though also used for colds and flus, tend to be primarily used for urinary tract and uric acid problems (like Joe Pye weed, gravel root). Interesting also is the traditional use of boneset (and many of the *Eupatorium* species) for snakebite as an antivenin throughout the world. Echinacea is also used in this manner, and like echinacea, boneset stimulates phagocytosis: the number and aggressiveness of white blood cells in the blood.

Clinical trials have shown that boneset stimulates phagocytosis better than echinacea, is analgesic (at least as effective as aspirin), and reduces cold and flu symptoms. In mice it has shown strong immunostimulant activity and cytotoxic action against cancer cells.

Increasing numbers of practicing herbalists report that boneset is a reliable and effective immunostimulant, *especially in infections that just*

> ## Things to Know about Boneset
>
> Boneset is unpleasantly bitter to most people. It can cause vomiting if large doses are taken hot, so care is indicated unless that is your desire.
>
> It is inexpensive and a reliable alternative and better for most of the things for which echinacea is wrongly prescribed. The homeopathic tincture (6x) has been found in human trials to be exceptionally effective in the treatment of colds and flus. During the nineteenth century, few farmhouses did not have bundles of boneset hung from the rafters for use at the first onset of chills and fever.

won't go away. So, if you are sick with a feverish disease with aching bones, get almost well, then relapse over and over again, feel weak and debilitated, and have a sense of mental unreality, boneset is indicated. It seems to be much better than echinacea for upper respiratory infections that have progressed to full-blown disease.

Preparation and Dosage

Boneset may be taken as tea or tincture.

Tea: *Cold:* 1 ounce (25 g) of herb in 1 quart (1 l) boiling water, let steep overnight, strain and drink throughout day. The cold infusion is for the mucous membrane system and is a liver tonic. *Hot:* 1 teaspoon herb in 8 ounces (237 ml) hot water, steep 15 minutes. Take 4 to 6 ounces (118 to 177 ml) up to 4 times per day. *Note:* boneset is only a diaphoretic when hot and should be consumed hot for active infections, chills, and fevers.

Tincture: Use fresh herb in flower 1:2 with 95 percent alcohol, use 20 to 40 drops up to 3 times day in hot water. *Dry herb:* 1:5 with 60 percent alcohol, use 30 to 50 drops in hot water up to 3 times a day. In acute viral or bacterial upper respiratory infections, use 10 drops of tincture in hot water every half hour up to 6 times a day. In chronic conditions when the acute stage has passed but there is continued chronic fatigue and relapse, use 10 drops of tincture in hot water 4 times a day.

Side Effects and Contraindications

The hot infusion in quantity can cause vomiting; otherwise, there are no side effects. It has been reported that the fresh plant contains trematol, which causes "milk-sickness" in cows and in people who drink infected milk. My research shows that trematol is confined to *Eupatorium rugosum,* white snakeroot, and does not occur in boneset. A significant number of clinicians feel that as a tincture, fresh boneset is best, and that the dried herb should be used for tea.

Alternatives to Boneset

Echinacea, licorice.

RED ROOT (*Ceanothus* spp.)

Family: Rhamnaceae.

Part used: The root.

Collection: In the fall or early spring, whenever the root has been subjected to a good frost. The inner bark of the root is a bright red, and this color extends through the white woody root as a pink tinge after a freeze. The root is extremely tough when it dries. It should be cut into small 1- or 2-inch pieces with plant snips while still fresh.

Actions: First and foremost a lymph system stimulant, anti-inflammatory, and tonic. It is also astringent, a mucous membrane tonic, alterative, antiseptic, expectorant, antispasmodic, and a blood coagulant.

Active against: I have been unable to find any studies testing *Ceanothus* against specific disease organisms. However, the historical record shows a long history of use for stubborn or fetid ulceration of the skin and mucous membranes, strep throat, general throat and upper respiratory infections, malaria, and diphtheria. Like oak (which has been found effective against numerous disease organisms), it is strongly astringent. There is every indication that *Ceanothus* will prove specific against particular disease organisms in spite of the dearth of scientific study.

About Red Root

Red root is an important herb in that it helps facilitate clearing of dead cellular tissue from the lymph system. When the immune system responds to acute conditions or the onset of disease, as white blood cells kill invading bacteria they are taken to the lymph system for disposal. When the lymph system can clear out dead cellular material rapidly, the healing process is increased, sometimes dramatically. The herb shows especially strong action whenever any portion of the lymph system is swollen, infected, or inflamed. This includes lymph nodes, tonsils (entire back of throat), spleen, and appendix. There is some evidence that the activity of red root in the lymph nodes also enhances the lymph nodes' production of lymphocytes, specifically the formation of T cells.

I have found that the action of echinacea increases dramatically when it is combined with red root or with red root and licorice. Historically, red root has also been considered specific for liver inflammation and congestion, and it may be of benefit in those conditions.

Preparation and Dosages

Red root is used as tincture, tea, strong decoction, gargle, or capsules.

Tincture: Dry root, 1:5 with 50 percent alcohol, 30 to 90 drops up to 4 times a day.

Tea: 1 teaspoon powdered root in 8 ounces (237 ml) water, simmer 15 minutes, strain. Drink up to 6 cups per day.

Strong decoction: 1 ounce (25 g) herb in 16 ounces (473 ml) water, simmer slowly 30 minutes covered. One tablespoon (15 ml) 3 or 4 times per day.

Gargle: In tonsillitis or throat inflammations, gargle with strong tea 4 to 6 times per day.

Capsules: 10 to 30 double-ought capsules per day.

Side Effects and Contraindications

No side effects have ever been noted. However, Michael Moore suggests caution by people using blood coagulants and advises against the use of large doses in pregnancy, because of its astringent action.

Alternatives to Red Root

Any red root species. One species, *Ceanothus thrysiflorus* (California lilac), has historically been successful in the treatment of malignant diphtheria. Other alternatives: cleavers, which is much milder (a food herb), poke root, which is much stronger (a drug herb) and should be used with care.

Identifying Red Root in the Wild

Red root can be a low-lying shrub or a tallish bush. The only thing that is reliably similar between species are the unique tiny, triangular seed pods. When ripe they are the same color as the tincture: a brilliant burgundy red. It is pervasive in its range. All species can be used interchangeably. It is a potent and useful member of any herbal repertory and one of my "if I could only choose ten herbs" list.

❀SIBERIAN GINSENG *(Eleutherococcus senticosus)*

Family: Araliaceae.

Part used: The root.

Collection: The plant is indigenous to northeast Asia but is now being grown commercially in a few places in the United States. It is usually commercially purchased, the root already cut and sifted to industry standards.

Actions: Adaptogen, antistressor, immune tonic, immunpotentiating (phagocytosis), immunoadjuvant (B lymphocytes), increases non-specific resistance against several pathogens, monoamine oxidase inhibitor.

Active against: I have found no specific activity for Siberian ginseng; however, it has been shown to increase nonspecific resistance in human beings against numerous pathogens.

About Siberian Ginseng

This herb, though used in China for several thousand years, was brought to prominence by intensive Russian research in the latter half of the twentieth century. Several clinical trials have shown significant immune-enhancing activity. This includes a significant increase in immunocompetent cells, specifically T lymphocytes (helper/inducer, cytotoxic, and natural killer cells). Tests of the herb have repeatedly shown that it increases the ability of human beings to withstand adverse conditions, increases mental alertness, and improves performance. People taking the herb regularly report fewer illnesses than those not taking it.

Siberian ginseng is, in general, completely nontoxic, and the Russians have reported people using exceptionally large doses for up to 20 years with no adverse reactions. Both Asian and American ginseng, on the other hand, do have several limitations on their use. Siberian ginseng, in my experience, produces cumulative results: the longer you use it, the better it works. It tends to kick in after 6 weeks or so, and the most significant results can be seen after 6 months of use. This is especially true in people with pale unhealthy skin, lassitude, and depression.

Siberian ginseng is specifically indicated for people with immunodepression, fatigue, and a lack of vitality and perhaps those who get sick a lot. Unlike echinacea, it is not an immune stimulant; rather, it is an immune enhancer and helps restore optimum functioning in the immune system. As it is a monoamine oxidase inhibitor, it is also useful in depression, a condition that often accompanies a severely depleted immune system.

Preparation and Dosage

Siberian ginseng is used as tea, as tincture, or in capsules.

Tea: Cold infusion, 3 to 6 ounces (85 to 170 g) up to 3 times a day.

Tincture: Dry herb 1:5 with 60 percent alcohol, 20 to 60 drops up to 3 times a day.

Capsules: 2 double-ought capsules 3 times a day.

Side Effects and Contraindications

For almost all people: none. May temporarily increase blood pressure in some people; blood pressure tends to drop to normal within a few weeks. Caution should be exercised by people with very high blood pressure, especially if the herb is combined with other hypertensives such as licorice. With extreme overuse: tension and insomnia.

Alternatives to Siberian Ginseng

Ashwagandha, astragalus, shiitake; for men over 40, Asian or American ginseng.

Caution for Those under Forty

Siberian ginseng is *the* ginseng to be used by anyone under 40 years of age. In general, neither American nor Asian ginseng should be used by young people, especially men under 40. Those ginsengs possess strong androgenic effects, and consistent use can interfere with sexual development. However, they are definitely indicated for anyone over 40. They have shown reliable antifatigue, antitumor, radioprotective, antiviral, and antioxidant activity. Those taking the herbs have consistently shown increased response to visual stimuli and increased alertness, power of concentration, and grasp of abstract concepts. Basically, these two ginsengs are herbs for those experiencing the side effects of aging. However, they are both very expensive. Siberian ginseng is an effective alternative unless there is accompanying sexual and/or mental debility, or for those with cancer and accompanying immune depression.

FOODS AND VITAMINS
FOR THE IMMUNE SYSTEM

Though we have already discussed the importance of garlic, ginger, and onions as herbal antibiotics, studies have shown that their regular use in the daily diet helps maintain the overall health of the body. Because garlic and ginger, and to a lesser extent onions, are active against all the major antibiotic-resistant bacteria and also enhance the healthy functioning of numerous systems in our bodies, it makes sense to include them in our food. Additionally, several vitamins have been found to be exceptionally important in immune health. The most important is vitamin C.

Benefits of Vitamin C

Vitamin C provides a protective function against free radicals, reduces wound healing time, supports strong connective tissue and coronary arteries, and seems to stimulate the immune system to remain strong and healthy. Human beings — all the higher primates, actually — are almost the only animals that cannot synthesize vitamin C in their bodies. This may partly explain the high numbers of plants rich in vitamin C (especially the evergreens) that were a regular part of the diet of indigenous peoples. Additionally, native peoples often used pine bark in conjunction with the fresh evergreen tips as medicine. Pine bark is higher than any other substance except grape seeds in proanthocyanidin, a powerful antioxidant and potentiator of vitamin C. Proanthocyanidin causes small amounts of vitamin C to produce the same effects in the body as significantly larger amounts.

Vitamin C is most effective when 1000 to 2000 milligrams are taken two to three times per day. It needs to be taken at least twice daily to keep it present in the body at necessary levels. At larger dosages it will cause flatulence and diarrhea, though the amount that produces this effect varies for each person. To find your dose level of vitamin C, take it in increasing amounts until the stools become soft, then reduce the amount slightly until they become

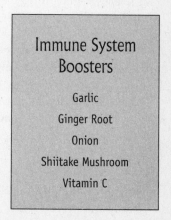

Immune System Boosters

Garlic

Ginger Root

Onion

Shiitake Mushroom

Vitamin C

firm. An effervescent form of the vitamin is one of the most pleasant forms for use. (Andrew Weil, in his *Eight Weeks to Optimum Health,* suggests the use of three additional vitamins: beta carotene with lycopene included [25,000 IU], vitamin E [400 IU under age 40, 800 IU over], and selenium [200 micrograms].)

SHIITAKE *(Lentinus edodes)*

Part used: The mushroom.

Collection: Mushrooms are a fruit, like apples. When they appear, before they begin to dry out, is the time to gather them. They are more commonly bought than found and have been a primary remedy in China for centuries.

Actions: Immunostimulant, antiviral, antitumor.

Active against: Viral encephalitis.

About Shiitake

Shiitake mobilizes the immune system against viruses, bacteria, cancer, and parasites. One of its major constituents, lentinan, has been shown to stimulate immunocompetent cells (T cell production and aggressiveness, natural killer cells, and macrophages), to be directly active against viral encephalitis, and to have potent antitumor activity, preventing metastasis of cancer to the lungs. In general, shiitake increases the activity and aggressiveness of the human immune system against abnormal cells and organisms defined as "not us."

Finding Shiitake Mushrooms

Shiitake is relatively easy to find in bulk at decent prices. The mushrooms can be bought dried in whole form and reconstituted for use as food or ground for encapsulation or use as a powder. The other two potent Asian mushrooms, maitake and reishi, are much harder to find. Maitake is also edible and can be found wild in the United States, where it is called hen of the woods. Maitake has the additional property of being active against HIV *in vitro*. Reishi is not edible, being a hard woody mushroom. Unfortunately, the commercial supplies of these two alternatives are limited, and they generally command unrealistic prices.

Immune Soup

Andrew Weil's recipe in Eight Weeks To Optimum Health *is the original inspiration for this potent immune soup. Like most cooks, I couldn't resist adding my two cents' worth. It is especially useful as fall turns to winter.*

      8 cups (237 ml) water
      1 tablespoon (15 ml) olive oil
      1 onion, diced
      1 bulb garlic (at least 10 cloves), minced
      One 1½-inch (3½ cm) piece of fresh gingerroot,
        grated
1½ cups salted vegebroth powder*
        (or vegetable soup stock, if desired)
      5 pieces sliced dried astragalus root
      2 cups fresh, sliced shiitake mushrooms
        (or 1 cup dried)
      1 large reishi mushroom
      Cayenne powder, if desired

1. Bring water to boil in large pot.
2. Heat olive oil, sauté garlic, onions, and ginger until soft and aromatic. Add contents of skillet to water. Add vegebroth powder, shiitake, astragalus, and reishi. Simmer covered two hours.
3. Remove from heat, allow to sit for two more hours.
4. Remove astragalus and reishi mushroom. Reheat.
5. Add salt and pepper to taste, and cayenne powder if desired (just enough so that it just brings out a light sweat).

*Available from Trinity Herb — see Resources

Preparation and Dosage

Shiitake mushrooms are generally used in capsules or as food.

Capsules: The capsules are usually commercially produced. Follow the manufacturer's directions. However, if you encapsulate your own, as a preventative use 2 double-ought capsules 2 times a day. In acute conditions, take up to 25 capsules per day.

Food: Eat as much and as often as desired (see sidebar on page 82).

Side Effects and Contraindications

None.

Alternatives to Shiitake

Reishi, maitake, cordyceps.

LIFESTYLE CHOICES

Though lifestyle choices are beyond the scope of this book, several of them significantly enhance immune functioning. They are sweat bathing or saunas at least once per month and more often when ill (in controlled trials, length and severity of illness has been reduced), moderate exercise (releases toxins from the body and works the lymph system), touching and massage (there is a direct correlation between being touched and immune health; additionally, massage stimulates lymph system functioning), positive thinking (if life is more fun to live, there is less unconscious desire to become ill), and diet (reducing commercial factory-farmed meats, increasing organic meats, and eating plants that have known effects on overall health).

4

MAKING AND USING HERBAL MEDICINES

In general, plants are used as medicines or made into medicines in five traditional ways: by infusing the herb in water (as teas, infusions, decoctions, washes, beers, or steams), by infusing the herb in alcohol or an alcohol-and-water combination (tinctures, fluid extracts, and, when diluted, as washes or sprays), by transferring the power of the herb to an oil base (salves and oils), by using the plant itself (eaten whole, wound powders, in capsules, smoking, or smudging), or by distilling and using the essential oil of the plant.

There are, of course, other media in which herbs can be extracted for use as medicine; vinegar, glycerine, and honey are three very good ones. They all will extract the medicinal qualities of a plant to differing degrees. The whole herb, water, and alcohol are the strongest; glycerin and honey are next; and vinegar and oil are next. Glycerine and honey extractions are extremely useful for children because of the sweet taste.

MAKING INFUSIONS

An infusion is made by immersing an herb in either cold or hot, not boiling, water for an extended time. (Basically, a tea is a weak

> Each tree, each shrub, and herb, down even to the grasses and mosses, agreed to furnish a remedy for some one of the diseases [of humankind] and each said: "I shall appear to help man whenever he calls upon me in his need."
>
> *THE TEACHINGS OF THE CHEROKEE NATION*

infusion.) The water you use should be the purest you can find, *not* tap water. Rainwater, distilled water, or water from healthy wells or springs is best. Infusions should be kept only a maximum of 3 days if refrigerated, 1 or 2 days if not refrigerated.

Proportions and Steeping Time

Unless you are making a steam, hot infusions should be prepared in tightly covered jars to keep the volatile oils from rising off the infusion as steam. Herbs that have a strong essential oil or perfumey smell when the leaves are crushed are usually high in volatile oils. Quart or pint canning jars are very good, as they will not break from heat, and the screw cap allows them to be shaken if desired and keeps any volatile oils from floating off as steam. I usually like to leave infusions overnight. I prepare them before bed and then strain them out the next morning and drink them throughout the day.

The following guidelines for making hot infusions will work with most herbs.

Leaves: 1 ounce (25 g) herb per quart (l) of water. Steep 4 hours in hot water, tightly covered. Tougher leaves require longer steeping.

Flowers: 1 ounce (25 g) herb per quart (l) of water. Steep 2 hours in hot water, tightly covered. More fragile flowers require less time.

Seeds: 1 ounce (25 g) herb per pint (475 ml) of water. Steep 30 minutes in hot water, tightly covered. More fragrant seeds such as fennel need less time (15 minutes); rose hips need a longer time (3 to 4 hours).

Barks and roots: 1 ounce (25 g) herb per pint (475 ml) of water. Steep 8 hours in hot water, tightly covered. Some barks, such as slippery elm, need less time (1 to 2 hours).

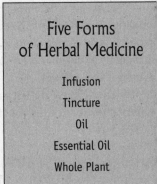

Five Forms of Herbal Medicine

Infusion

Tincture

Oil

Essential Oil

Whole Plant

Hot Infusion for Parasites

This is a traditional infusion used to eliminate intestinal worms. For malaria, it should be twice as strong, and the dosage doubled. It is very bitter.

> 2 ounces (57 g) dried wormwood leaves
>   (*Artemisia absinthium*)
> 2 quarts (2 l) water

1. Place wormwood in container, pour near-boiling water on top, cover tightly, and let sit overnight.
2. Strain, and press wormwood to remove as much liquid as possible.
To Use: Drink 1 cup (250 ml) 4 times per day. This amount will last 2 days. Make it again every 2 days, and continue for 8 days.

Cold Infusions

Cold infusions are preferable for some herbs. The bitter components of herbs tend to be less water soluble. Yarrow, for instance, is much less bitter when prepared in cold water. Cold infusions usually need to steep for much longer periods of time. Each herb is different.

MAKING DECOCTIONS

Decoctions, prepared with boiling, can be much more potent than infusions and are generally prepared for use as compresses, enemas, and syrups. Like infusions, decoctions should be kept only for a maximum of 3 days if refrigerated, 1 or 2 days if not refrigerated.

Proportions and Boiling Time

The standard pharmaceutical approach to decoctions is 1 ounce (25 g) of herb per pint (475 ml) of water boiled for 15 minutes and strained when cool; water is then added to bring the total volume back to 1 pint. I approach the process a little differently: I take 1 ounce (25 g) of herb in 3 cups (750 ml) of water and boil slowly and steadily until the liquid is reduced to one half. (If larger amounts of the decoction are desired, the amounts of water and herb may be increased.) The boiling should take place in a stainless steel or glass container, never aluminum.

The doses can range from a tablespoon to a cup depending on the plant used. For use as a compress, you simply soak a sterile bandage in the decoction and then place it on the body. As a syrup, add honey to taste.

Decoction for Colds and Flu

1 ounce (25 g) dried leaves of white or
   culinary sage
3 cups (750 ml) water
Honey
Juice of 1 lemon
Cayenne

1. Boil sage at a slow boil in 3 cups (750 ml) water until liquid is reduced by one half. Let cool.
2. Strain liquid, and press sage to remove as much liquid as possible.
3. Reheat to barely hot, and add fresh wildflower honey to taste. Let cool; add juice of 1 lemon and a pinch of cayenne.
4. Store in refrigerator.
To Use: Take 1 tablespoon (15 ml) (cold) to 1 cup (250 ml) (hot) as often as needed for the beginning of throat or upper respiratory infections.

MAKING STEAMS AND WASHES

Steams and washes are other easy ways to extract the properties of herbs into water. Steams are especially excellent for upper respiratory infections. They can be used as often as desired or needed. Wonderful steams are made from eucalyptus, juniper, or sage, as in the following recipe.

This recipe can also be used as a wash for wounds. Rather than boiling, bring it to the edge of boiling, remove from heat, and let steep until lukewarm. Wash wound thoroughly and then apply wound powder (see page 96).

Steam for Upper Respiratory Infections

This recipe can be prepared with fresh herbs or essential oils if desired. To substitute essential oils, add 30 drops each of essential oils of rosemary, sage, juniper, eucalyptus, or bergamot to 1 quart (1 l) of water.

2 ounces (57 g) young eucalyptus leaves, dried
1 ounce (25 g) sage leaf, dried
1 ounce (25 g) juniper leaf or berry, dried
1 gallon (4 l) water

1. Place herbs in water (in glass, stainless steel, or ceramic-coated pot) and bring to rolling boil.
2. Remove from heat, hold head over steam, and cover head and steaming pot with large towel. Breathe steam deep into lungs.
3. Return to heat and bring herbs to a boil again to repeat as often as necessary. Add fresh herbs when their strong smell begins to noticeably diminish.

MAKING AN ALCOHOL TINCTURE

A tincture is made by immersing a fresh or dried plant in full-strength alcohol or an alcohol and water mixture. Alcohol is extractive: it pulls all the water out of plants into itself. The resulting tincture is a mix of both water and alcohol. With fresh plants, the liquid tincture is generally equal to the amount of liquid added at the beginning. With dried plant material, especially roots, the final volume is often much less than what you started with.

Store tinctures in amber jars out of the sun. Alcohol-based tinctures will generally last for many years. Because of the shelf life and ease of dispensing, many herbalists prefer tinctures over capsules and infusions. Tinctures from various herbs can be combined for dispensing as a blend (although a certain few such as myrrh and propolis do not combine well).

Using Fresh Herbs

Fresh leafy plants may be chopped or left whole before placing them into the alcohol or pureed with the alcohol in a blender. Fresh roots should be ground with the alcohol in a blender into a pulpy mush. Fresh plants naturally contain a certain percentage of water. When a tincture is made from fresh plants the plant is placed in 190 proof alcohol (95 percent alcohol): one part plant to two parts alcohol. For example, if you have 3 ounces (85 g) (dry measure) of fresh echinacea flower heads, they would be placed in a jar with 6 ounces (177 ml) (liquid measure) of 190 proof alcohol.

I generally use well-sealed Mason jars, store out of the sun, and shake daily. At the end of 2 weeks, decant the herb and squeeze in a cloth until as dry as possible (an herb or wine press is good for this), and store the resulting liquid in labeled amber bottles.

Using Dried Herbs

Plants as they dry lose their natural moisture content. Some plants, like myrrh gum, contain virtually none; others, like mint, contain a great deal. When making a tincture of a dried plant you add back the amount of water that was present in the plant when it was fresh. Many books list the amount of water that should be added back. One good one, and the one I use, is Michael Moore's *Herbal Materia Medica* listed in the Resources. Generally dried plants are tinctured at a 5:1 ratio, that is, five parts liquid to one part dried herb. For example, echinacea root contains 30 percent water by weight. If you have 10 ounces (284 g) of powdered echinacea root you would add to it 50 ounces (1479 ml) of liquid (1:5), of which 35 ounces (1035 ml) is 95 percent alcohol and 15 ounces (444 ml) is water. Again, do not use tap water. Dried herbs are generally powdered as fine as possible, usually in a blender or Vita-mix. It is best to store herbs as whole as possible until they are needed. The tincture is left for 2 weeks and then decanted.

Combination Tincture Formula for Colds and Flu

This blend will usually prevent the onset of colds and flu for people with relatively healthy immune systems.

⅓ ounce (10 ml) echinacea tincture
⅓ ounce (10 ml) red root tincture
⅓ ounce (10 ml) licorice tincture

Combine the three tinctures in a 1-ounce (30 ml) amber bottle with a dropper.
To Use: Take a dropper full (30 drops) at least each hour during the onset of upper respiratory infections.

Making Nasal Sprays from Tinctures

Nasal sprays are excellent for helping with the onset of upper respiratory or sinus infections. Simply take an herbal tincture and place up to 10 drops or so in a nasal spray bottle (available from pharmacies). Add pure water and spray up nostrils as often as needed. Two drops each of the essential oils of eucalyptus, juniper, sage, and rosemary may be substituted for the tinctures.

Nasal Spray Formula for Sinus Infections

5 drops eucalyptus tincture
5 drops usnea tincture
5 drops echinacea tincture
5 drops sage tincture
5 drops juniper tincture
3 drops grapefruit seed extract

Place tinctures in a 1-ounce (30 ml) nasal spray bottle, add pure water to make 1 ounce (30 ml), and replace cap.
To Use: Spray into nostrils as often as desired.

MAKING OIL INFUSIONS

Oil infusions are exceptionally useful for burns, sunburn, chapped and dry skin, skin infections, and ear drops and for use on wounds as salves. The medicinal properties of the plant are transferred to an oil base. For a salve, the oil is made thick and moderately hard by adding beeswax.

Using Dried Herbs

To make an oil infusion of *dried* herbs, take the herbs you wish to use and grind them into as fine a powder as possible. Place the herbs in a glass baking dish and cover with oil. Olive oil is a good choice because it is the one oil that will not go rancid; it is strongly antimicrobial. Stir the herbs to make sure they are well saturated with oil, then add just enough oil to cover them by ½ to ¼ inch (13 to 6¼ mm). You may leave them in the sun for 2 weeks or bake them in the oven on the lowest heat your oven allows for 8 hours or overnight. Some herbalists prefer to simmer the herbs and oil for as many as 10 days at 100°F (38°C) in a slow cooker. When the preparation is ready, strain the oil out of the herbs by pressing in a strong cloth with a tight weave.

Using Fresh Herbs

To make an oil infusion from *fresh* herbs, place the herbs in a Mason jar and cover them with just enough oil to leave no part of the plant is exposed to air. Let sit in the sun for 2 weeks, or cook in a Crock-Pot for 5 days at low setting. Then press the herbs through a cloth. Let the decanted oil sit. After a day, the water naturally present in the herbs will settle to the bottom. Pour off the oil and discard the water. Some herbalists prefer to start the oil infusion by letting the herb sit in just a bit of alcohol that has been poured over the leaves for 24 hours. This breaks down the cell walls of the plant and helps begin the extraction process. After this, add the oil and proceed as above.

Herbal Oil for Skin Infections

Oils are exceptionally good for the health and healing of the skin.

1 quart (1 l) olive oil
1 ounce (25 g) usnea
1 ounce (25 g) acacia
1 ounce (25 g) echinacea root or seed
1 ounce (25 g) garlic
1 ounce (25 g) sage

1. Add the oil to a heavy pot. Use glass or stainless steel, not aluminum or cast iron.
2. Grind all the herbs as fine as possible.
3. Add the herbs to the oil.
4. Heat the mixture overnight in the oven with the setting on low (150° to 200°F [66° to 93°C]), or heat covered on low in a Crock-Pot for 7 days.
5. Remove the pot from the oven and let the mixture cool. Press the oily herb mixture through a cloth to extract the oil.
6. Store the oil in a sealed glass container out of the sun. It does not need to be refrigerated.

Formula for a Good Wound Salve

      1 quart (1 l) olive oil
    ¾ ounce (21 g) echinacea, seeds or root, ground fine
      1 ounce (25 g) cryptolepsis root, ground fine
  1½ ounces (43 g) juniper, ground fine
      1 ounce (25 g) oak bark or krameria or wild
        geranium, ground fine
      1 ounce (25 g) acacia leaf
    ½ ounce (14 g) wormwood, powdered
    ½ ounce (14 g) usnea, powdered
      4 ounces (113 g) beeswax
    ¼ teaspoon (1 ml) vitamin E
    ¼ teaspoon (1 ml) eucalyptus essential oil

1. Make an oil infusion by combining all the herbs with olive oil (see page 92.)
2. Add the herbal oil infusion back to the pot used to make the infusion and reheat it slowly on the stovetop.
3. Measure out the beeswax and add to the pot. A good estimate is 2 ounces (57 g) of wax to every pint (475 ml) of infused oil (so for this formula, about 4 ounces [113 g]). Many people like the beeswax grated, but I just break it up into small pieces. Heat until beeswax is melted.
4. Remove pan from stove. Let mixture cool until just before it starts to harden, then add vitamin E oil and eucalyptus essential oil, and stir well.
5. While mixture is still liquid, pour into salve containers and label. *Note:* Make sure your containers are made to withstand hot liquids before using them.

Making a Salve

A salve is really just an oil hardened with beeswax. Make an oil infusion, then put it into a glass or stainless steel cooking pan. Heat it gently on top of the stove. Add chopped beeswax to the warmed oil, usually 2 ounces (57 g) per cup (250 ml) of oil. When the beeswax is melted, place a few drops from the pot on a small plate, let it cool, and touch it. If it is too soft, add more wax; if too hard, add a bit more oil. A perfect salve should stay hard for a few seconds as you press your finger tip on it, then suddenly soften from your body heat. I used to pour my salves into hundreds of tiny salve containers, but now I just pour the whole batch into a Mason jar. If I want to put some into a small salve jar for use, I heat it in the oven or microwave until it liquifies.

PREPARATIONS FROM WHOLE HERBS

Some wounds do not respond well to a wet dressing like a salve. In that case, I use powdered herbs directly on the wound. Herbal wound powders, ground fine, stop bleeding and facilitate rapid healing while preventing infection. After the wound has begun to heal, switching to a wound salve continues that process. There is probably no more powerful way to treat skin infections than with powdered herbs. I have yet to find a wound infection that will not respond to one.

Eating the Herb

Many herbs can be harvested and eaten in whole form. Wormwood root, a prime example, can be used for sore throats and upper respiratory infections of both viral and bacterial origin. It is very strong, and a bit of fresh root can be carried in the pocket and a little eaten whenever needed. Sometimes a combination of whole herbs and tinctured herbs works well; in this instance, wormwood root with a supportive combination of echinacea, red root, and licorice tincture for upper respiratory infections.

Powders and Capsules

Capsules are good for getting a large quantity of herb in whole form into the body. The herb must be powdered as finely as possible and then

Wound Powder

1 ounce (25 g) goldenseal root
1 ounce (25 g) usnea
1 ounce (25 g) echinacea root or seed
1 ounce (25 g) eucalyptus leaf
1 ounce (25 g) juniper leaf

1. Powder all herbs as fine as possible. Usually I begin with a Vita-mix and then move the powder to a nut or coffee grinder for further powdering.
2. After the herbs have been powdered, sift through a fine mesh sieve.
3. Store this powder in the freezer or in a securely closed container and out of the sunlight. Powdered herbs lose their potency fairly quickly unless protected. At the least, this mixture should be replaced every 6 months unless it is frozen; in that case, at minimum every year.
To Use: When the powder is needed, sprinkle it liberally on wet wounds. It will stop the bleeding, prevent infection, and stimulate cell wall binding. Infected, oozing, pus-filled wounds should be opened up and cleaned, and the powder liberally sprinkled on as often as needed. Once the wound is healing cleanly it should not be disturbed (i.e., by scrubbing or trying to open it up again); just add more wound powder as needed.

This same formula can be sprinkled onto feet or into shoes and socks for athlete's foot fungal infections. It may also be used on babies for diaper rash.

encapsulated — a tedious process. I usually try to bribe my son to do it or just buy it ready-made from a retail source. Goldenseal is an excellent herb for use in capsules. Sometimes the herbs are powdered and *not* encapsulated. For instance, with stomach ulceration the herbs should be powdered, mixed with liquid, and consumed. This allows the herb to make contact with the entire affected area. If the ulceration is in the duodenum, which lies just below the stomach, then capsules would be used. The capsules tend to sit at the bottom of the stomach and then drop through into the duodenum, where they are needed. Duodenal ulcers are often accompanied by painful cramping or spasming. This can be alleviated by the addition of a few drops of peppermint essential oil to the herbal mixture before encapsulating it.

Caution

As with all medicines, it is important with both adults and children to pay close attention to how they respond to herbs. Start with small doses and work up. At any sign of adverse reactions, the herb should be discontinued. If severe symptoms persist, consult a competent health care provider.

USING ESSENTIAL OILS

Essential oils are made by distilling volatile oils from plants. Essential oil makes up ½ to 5 percent of a plant's weight, most plants tending toward the lower end of the scale. For a plant that is 1 percent essential oil, it will take 100 ounces of plant (a little over 6 pounds [2¾ kg]) to get 1 ounce (30 ml) of essential oil.

Knowledge of herbal medicine was considered exceptionally important for prospective wives and mothers during the Middle Ages, and few homes did not have their own "still rooms" where herbal medicines were prepared. Distilling plant essences was a part of this herbal knowledge for many women, and aromatherapy had its birth in rudimentary form in Europe at that time. Most people buy their essential oils, but I have met a few wise women who are reclaiming this long-lost tradition and are distilling their own essences from the plants that grow in the fields and valleys near their homes. Most of us, however, buy them ready-made.

Five-Step Herbal Regimen for an Ulcerated Stomach

4 ounces (113 g) dried licorice root
4 ounces (113 g) dried comfrey root
Ninety 300 mg bismuth capsules
1 ounce (30 ml) grapefruit seed extract
2 ounces (59 ml) eucalyptus tincture
2 ounces (59 ml) goldenseal tincture
2 ounces (59 ml) acacia tincture
1 quart (1 l) wildflower honey

1. Powder licorice and comfrey root as fine as possible, and mix together in equal parts. Take 2 tablespoons (30 ml) twice a day (morning and evening), mixed in any liquid of choice (e.g., apple juice), for 30 days. For the next 60 days, use 1 tablespoon (15 ml) licorice (or marshmallow) root mornings only. The herbs should not be in capsules in order to allow them to fully coat the stomach lining. (For duodenal ulcers, take in capsules.)

2. Take 300 mg bismuth 3 times a day for 30 days (or Pepto-bismol in similar quantities). This has been found to facilitate ulcer healing time.

3. Take 6 drops grapefruit seed extract 3 times a day for 15 days. Place it in a small glass of orange or grapefruit juice — it is too bitter for anything else.

4. Mix 2 ounces (59 ml) each of eucalyptus, goldenseal, and acacia tinctures. Take 1 teaspoon (5 ml) of the tincture 3 times a day for 15 days.

5. Take 1 tablespoon (15 ml) honey 6 times a day for 30 days.

Essential oils work by directly making contact with bacteria that reside on the mucous membranes of the nose and sinuses and by absorption through those mucous linings directly into the system. In this way the active principles of the plant bypass the gastrointestinal tract, and go directly into the bloodstream. Because it takes so much of a plant to make an essential oil, these oils are very strong in their actions. To get an idea of their strength: by taking a whole ounce of essential oil into the body (a bad idea, by the way), you would essentially be consuming 6 pounds (2¾ kg) of a plant in a form that would go to work in the body nearly instantly. That is why essential oils are greatly diluted, used in diffusers, or taken internally in minute doses (from 1 to 5 drops at a time). They can be extremely toxic when taken internally.

Common Applications

One of the best ways to use essential oils is in a diffuser, which diffuses the essential oil into the room air of homes or offices so that the healing properties of the plant can be breathed in throughout the day. Diffusers come in many styles; the best are electric, with a small air compressor that breaks up the essential oil into tiny droplets and spreads them out into the air. Follow the instructions that come with the diffuser.

Essential Oil Mix for Airborne Infections

1 ounce (30 ml) bergamot essential oil
1 ounce (30 ml) lavender essential oil
1 ounce (30 ml) eucalyptus essential oil
1 ounce (30 ml) distilled water

Combine all essential oils in a glass bottle. Add 10 to 12 drops of the essential oil blend to 1 ounce (30 ml) distilled water, and shake well.
To Use: Add oil blend to a diffuser.

Essential oils can also be taken in nasal sprays, added to hot water and inhaled, and used in sweat lodges or saunas. A few can be taken internally if caution is exercised. Some essential oils, such as wormwood, are so strong that internal use is not recommended under any conditions. Essential oils are best used internally under the direction of a qualified aromatherapist.

PREPARATIONS FOR COMMON CHILDREN'S AILMENTS

Ear infections are a significant problem among young children, especially those in day care. Day care centers, like hospitals, are one of the strongest breeding grounds for antibiotic-resistant bacteria, which are rapidly passed back and forth in the student population.

A significant number of studies have found that children who are treated for ear infections with antibiotics, surgery, and pharmaceutical decongestants have far higher numbers of ear infections throughout childhood and, in the case of surgical interventions, far higher problems with hearing loss than other children. Several studies have shown that children who receive *no* treatment at all, even for severe ear infections, fare far better in the long run than children who receive medical intervention.

Preventing Ear Infections

Here are several things to keep in mind to ensure children's health and minimize ear infections:
- Bottle-fed babies and small children have a higher incidence of ear infections than those who are breast fed.
- Babies and children who lie on their backs when drinking from a bottle tend to have a far higher incidence of ear infections (the milk sometimes runs into the ear canal). It is much better to hold them in your arms with their heads higher than their body or, if they can sit, to drink sitting up.
- Dairy products in the diet contribute significantly to the incidence of ear infections.

- Children experience many minor infections early in life as part of building their immunity to infectious diseases. In most instances, the immune system adjusts and the disease passes. As part of this process, children in day care will get significantly more infections than children who stay home.
- Dietary and herbal care will, in most instances, take care of the majority of childhood ear infections.
- Breast feeding, natural childbirth, frequent touching, and colonization of the baby's body with the mother's body bacteria immediately after birth will create the strongest immune system for the child and minimize childhood ear infections.
- For babies who are still being breast fed, if the mother takes doses of herbs herself at the level for treating acute upper respiratory infections, they will come out in the breast milk and go from there into the baby's system.
- For the very young, glycerites or medicinal honeys are of great benefit, as most babies and small children like them immensely.

> ## Caution
>
> The digestive system of children under one year old has not formed enough to protect itself from botulism organisms sometimes found in raw, uncooked honey. The Centers for Disease Control recommends that raw honey not be given to children under one year old as it can cause a sometimes fatal diarrhea. After one year the digestive and immune systems are able to protect the child from the organism. You should exercise caution in giving honey to younger children.

Treating Childhood Ear Infections

Most childhood ear infections can be treated successfully by using an herbal ear oil; eliminating all dairy products; drinking herbal teas; eating immune soup throughout the duration of the illness; using appropriate herbal tinctures, honeys, or glycerites; and using herbal steams.

Children are most susceptible to ear infections from antibiotic-resistant strains of *Haemophilus influenzae, Staphylococcus aureus, Streptococcus pneumoniae,* and *Branhamella catarrhalis.* The above treatment plan has been found highly effective for treating such infections.

Oil for Ear Infection

5 cloves garlic
4 ounces (118 ml) olive oil
20 drops essential oil of eucalyptus
15 drops grapefruit seed extract

1. Chop garlic fine, place in small baking dish with olive oil and bake in oven at lowest setting you have overnight.
2. Strain oil in a cloth, and press well.
3. Add essential oil of eucalyptus and grapefruit seed extract to garlic oil, and mix well.
4. Place in amber bottle for storage.
To Use: Hold glass eye dropper under hot water for 1 minute, dry well (quickly), and suction up oil from bottle. Place 2 drops in each ear every half hour or as often as needed.

Ear Infection Tincture Combination

You can also prepare this recipe as a glycerite or a medicinal honey (see page 104).

1 ounce (30 ml) ginger tincture
1 ounce (30 ml) echinacea tincture
1 ounce (30 ml) red root tincture
1 ounce (30 ml) licorice tincture

Combine the tinctures in one bottle and mix well.
To Use: Give 1 full dropper (30 drops) of the tincture each hour per 150 pounds (68 kg) of body weight until symptoms cease. Best administered in juice. (See page 103 for children's dosages.)

Brigitte Mars's Herb Tea for Ear Infections

1 ounce (25 g) Mormon tea *(Ephedra nevadensis)*
1 ounce (25 g) rose hips
1 ounce (25 g) elder flowers (*Sambucus* spp.)
1 ounce (25 g) licorice root
1 ounce (25 g) peppermint leaves
1 quart (1 l) water

1. Roughly crush all herbs.
2. Pour near-boiling water over herbs and steep until cool enough to drink. Consume as hot as is comfortable for drinking. Sweeten with honey if desired.
To Use: As much as is wanted can be consumed. The Mormon tea is a decongestant, the rose hips are slightly astringent, anti-inflammatory, and high in vitamin C, the elder flowers are slightly sedative and reduce fevers, the licorice root is anti-inflammatory, tastes good, and is antiviral and antibacterial, and the peppermint helps reduce fevers, decongests, and is calming. Catnip can be added to help lower fever.

DETERMINING PROPER DOSAGE FOR CHILDREN

Children are much smaller than adults and are generally more sensitive to herbs. Dosages should be adjusted when making herbal medicines for children by using one of these three common approaches:

Clark's Rule: Divide the weight in pounds by 150 to give an approximate fraction of an adult's dose. For a 75-pound (34 kg) child the dose would be 75 divided by 150, or ½ the adult dose.

Cowling's Rule: The child's age at his or her next birthday divided by 24. For a child approaching 8 years, the dose would be 8 divided by 24, or ⅓ the adult dose.

Young's Rule: The child's age divided by (12 + age of child). For a 3-year-old, it would be 3 divided by (12 + 3), or 15, for a dose of ⅕ the adult dose.

Making Herbal Glycerites and Honeys

Glycerites and honeys are excellent for children because of their wonderful taste. (See caution box on page 101.) Additionally, honey as an herbal medium adds honey's powerful actions to that of the herb. When making glycerites, use only food-grade vegetable glycerine or organic wildflower honey.

Using dry herbs: 1 part herb to 5 parts liquid, liquid composed of 10 percent 95 percent alcohol, 60 percent glycerin or honey, 30 percent water. So if you have 5 ounces (142 g) of well-powdered echinacea root or goldenseal, you would want 25 ounces (739 ml) of liquid of which 2½ ounces (75 ml) would be 95 percent alcohol, 15 ounces (444 ml) would be glycerine or honey, and 7½ ounces (222 ml) would be water. Mix all liquids well, add powdered dry herb, and leave in capped Mason jar for 2 weeks, shaking daily. Decant, and squeeze herb in cloth to extract as much liquid as possible. Store the glycerite or honey in an amber bottle out of the sun.

Using fresh herbs: Use 1 part herb to 2 parts liquid: 15 percent 95 percent alcohol and 85 percent glycerine or honey. So if you have 5 ounces (142 g) fresh herb, you would want 10 ounces (296 ml) of liquid, of which 1½ ounces (44 ml) would be 95 percent alcohol and 8½ ounces (251 ml) would be glycerine or honey.

Dosage: Generally, glycerites and honeys are not as strong as tinctures and may be given at 1½ times the dosage of tinctures. If you would normally give ½ dropper (15 drops) you could give ¾ dropper (22 drops).

Easing Fever and Diarrhea

Children are susceptible to diarrheal infections from the fearsome *E. coli* O157:H7 and antibiotic-resistant strains of *Shigella dyseneriae*. When they get extremely ill with these bacteria they may also experience high fever.

The best herb for lowering seriously high fevers is coral root *(Corallorhiza maculata),* either as a tea or as a tincture: 1 teaspoon of the root steeped in 8 ounces (236 ml) water for 30 minutes and drunk, or up to 30 drops tincture for a child of 60 pounds (27 kg). Brigitte Mars's Herb Tea on the previous page, with the addition of 1 ounce (30 ml) catnip, is also exceptionally effective in lowering fevers. Finally, bathing the child with washcloths soaked in cool water is highly effective.

For diarrhea, a tea and tincture combination is usually effective.

Rosemary Gladstar's Tea for Diarrhea

3 parts blackberry root
2 parts slippery elm bark

1. Mix the herbs together (for example, 3 ounces [85 g] blackberry root and 2 ounces [57 g] slippery elm bark).
2. Simmer 1 teaspoon of the herb mixture in 1 cup (250 ml) water for 20 minutes.
3. Strain and cool.
To Use: Take 2 to 4 tablespoons (30 to 60 ml) every hour, or as often as needed.

Tincture Combination for Diarrhea

1 ounce (30 ml) goldenseal root tincture
1 ounce (30 ml) acacia tincture
1 ounce (30 ml) cryptolepsis tincture
⅓ ounce (10 ml) grapefruit seed extract

Combine tinctures, shake well.
To Use: Give full dropper (30 drops) for every 150 pounds (68 kg) of body weight every 1 to 2 hours in water or orange juice until symptoms cease. If symptoms persist longer than 48 hours, see a physician. The severe *E. coli* O157:H7 bacteria is quite dangerous, especially to children.

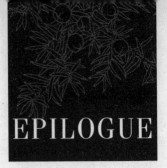

EPILOGUE

Underestimating the evolutionary potential of living organisms is the single most important mistake made by those who use chemical means to subdue nature.

MARC LAPPÉ, PH.D.

One of the most important lessons from our ancient legends and myths is that the gods take a dim view of human arrogance. Ancient versions of this message are to be found in the story of the woman who thought she could weave better than the gods and, after losing a weaving contest, was turned into a spider for her presumption. Another is the legend of Achilles, whose mother dipped him into water that made him invulnerable — except, of course, for the heel by which she held him. To this day, an "Achilles' heel" serves to remind us of the foolishness of thinking ourselves invulnerable. An even more recent warning to us is Mary Shelley's book *Frankenstein*. The message in her book was the same as that of the ancient legends and myths; in this instance, the warning was specifically about the arrogance of medical science in thinking it could take upon itself the capacities of the gods. In spite of our learning and great technology, these older warnings are still relevant to our species. As Vaclav Havel so eloquently put it, there are powers in the Universe against which it is advisable not to blaspheme. Perhaps it is fitting that the lowly bacteria will be the one to teach us humility.

Chymia egregia ancilla medicinae; non alia pejor domina.
(Chemistry makes an excellent handmaid but the worst possible mistress.)

GLOSSARY

Abortificant or Abortifacient: An agent that causes abortion, usually by increasing blood flow to the uterus. Sometimes a substance that causes deformation of the fetus, inducing the body to spontaneously abort.

Acute: An illness that comes on quickly, has severe symptoms, and a generally short duration, e.g., measles or colds. The opposite of chronic.

Allopathic: Conventional modern medicine. Originally only one of eight or so schools of medicine in the United States. By 1930, through a brilliant blend of legislative action, money generation through advertising in the *Journal of the American Medical Association*, control over the licensing of medical schools, and deceptive conciliation of other medical organizations, the allopaths gained complete control over American medicine. Prices and quality of health care suffered accordingly.

Alterative: Term not used in allopathic (or conventional) medicine that means a plant or procedure that stimulates physical changes in the body that will appropriately deal with chronic or acute diseases. A substance that renews tissues and improves function slowly and efficiently, culminating in health. Many herbs show their alterative aspect only in the presence of disease symptoms. In a healthy person, nothing or something entirely different happens.

Amenorrhea: Absence or abnormal cessation of menses.

Anaphrodisiac: Substance that depresses sexual desire and drive.

Analgesic: Substance that relieves pain without unconsciousness.

Anesthetic: Substance that decreases the capacity of nerves to experience pain.

Anodyne: Substance that eases pain.

Anthelmintic: Substance that is destructive to worms, usually taken internally.

Antibiotic: Substance that selectively depresses or destroys bacteria (literally "antilife").

Antibody: Entities in the cells and blood that actively attack and destroy disease pathogens.

Anticatarrhal: Catarrh is the inflammation of a mucous membrane, usually the air passages of the head or throat, with subsequent copious discharge of mucus. An anticatarrhal is a substance that reduces, prevents, or eliminates catarrh.

Anticoagulant: Substance that slows or stops the clotting of blood.

Antidepressant: Substance that counters depression or sadness.

Antifungal: Substance that kills or inhibits fungus.

Antihemorrhagic: A hemostatic.

Antihepatoxic: Substance that prevents toxins from negatively affecting the liver.

Antihypertensive: Substance that lowers blood pressure.

Anti-inflammatory: Substance that reduces inflammation.

Antimicrobial: Substance that inhibits or kills microorganisms.

Antimutagenic: Substance that reduces or interferes with mutagenic activity of other substances.

Antioxidant: Substance that slows or stops oxidation. In herbalism, specifically one that slows the formation of free-radicals.

Antipyretic: Substance that reduces fever.

Antirheumatic: Substance that eases, prevents, or reduces rheumatic symptoms.

Antiscorbutic: Substance that prevents scurvy, usually one that contains vitamin C.

Antiseptic: Substance that prevents putrefaction, the decay of cells, and infection.

Antispasmodic: Substance that relieves or prevents muscle spasms.

Antitussive: Substance that relieves or prevents cough.

Antiviral: Substance that kills viruses or inhibits their reproduction.

Aphrodisiac: An agent that increases sexual desire and drive.

Aperient: Substance that exerts a mild laxative activity.

Aromatic: Characteristic of herbs that have a strong, usually pleasant smell. Aromatic almost always refers to plants with volatile oils, usually ones that uplift the spirit, provide antibacterial action, or calm the nerves.

Arteriosclerosis: Condition of blood vessels that have thickened, hardened, lost their elasticity due to age or the buildup of fatty plaques along the vessel walls.

Arthritis: Inflammation of the joints. Either osteoarthritis (a degenerative bone disease involving loss and calcification of joint cartilage, so that the bones formerly cushioned by gristle now grind together, are painful, and become inflamed) or rheumatoid arthritis, a chronic and increasingly worsening inflammation of the joints from an unknown cause (believed to be an autoimmune condition).

Astringent: Substance that causes constriction of tissues. In herbal medicine, usually a plant that contains tannins, stops bleeding, and reduces inflammation. In any event, it dries out your mouth if you taste it.

Bitter tonic: Bitter-tasting substance that increases gastric secretions, tonifies the stomach, increases deficient appetite, and increases stomach acidity. These all aid deficient digestion.

Bronchitis: Inflammation of bronchial mucous membranes.

Candidiasis: Any disease condition caused by the yeast *Candida albicans*. It is commonly found on the skin and in the mouth, vagina, and rectum. Overuse of antibiotics and anti-inflammatory drugs, which interfere with the normal metabolic checks and balances of the body, has caused many people to suffer from candidiasis and allowed the once rare disease to become something of a national celebrity.

Cardiotonic: Substance that regulates or strengthens heart action and metabolism; whatever the condition of the heart, a cardiotonic brings it back to a normal range of action.

Carminative: An agent that aids the elimination of gas.

Cathartic: Substance that eases griping and expels gas.

Cholagogue: Substance that induces gallbladder contraction.

Choleretic: Substance that encourages the liver to produce bile.

Chronic: Disease that is of long, slow duration marked by general debility, sometimes with interspersed acute episodes. The opposite of acute.

Colitis: Inflammation of the colon.

Conjunctivitis: Inflammation of the mucous membranes of the eye or eyelid.

Counterirritant: Substance applied to the skin that produces an irritation, heating, or vasodilating action. Generally, it speeds healing by increasing blood circulation and warming deep (usually joint) inflammations.

Demulcent: Substance that reduces, relieves, or soothes irritation, particularly of mucous membrane surfaces.

Depurant: Substance that stimulates excretion.

Diaphoretic: Substance that increases perspiration.

Diuretic: Substance that increases the flow of urine.

Duodenum: The beginning of the small intestine; lies just below the stomach.

Dysmenorrhea: Painful menstruation.

Dyspepsia: Poor digestion, often with heartburn and stomach acid reflux.

Eczema: Chronic skin inflammation.

Emmenagogue: Substance that induces the onset of menses.

Emollient: Substance or herb that soothes, moistens, and lubricates the skin because of its mucilaginous compounds. (When used internally it is called a demulcent.)

Expectorant: Substance that causes mucus in the lungs and bronchial passages to come out more easily, usually through coughing.

Febrifuge: Substance that reduces fever.

Gastritis: Inflammation of the stomach lining.

Gout: Inflammation of joints caused by uric acid crystals lodging in them.

Hemostatic: Substance that either slows or stops bleeding.

Hepatic: Substance that acts on the liver.

Hepatitis: Inflammation of the liver.

Herb: Plant used for medicinal or culinary purposes.

Hiatus hernia: Protrusion of the stomach through a tear in the diaphragm wall.

Hypnotic: An herb that induces sleep.

Hypotensive: A substance that lowers blood pressure.

Immunostimulant: A substance that stimulates the immune system's health and ability to respond to disease either gradually or quickly.

Infusion: An extremely strong tea made with either hot or cold water and an herb.

In vitro: In a test tube.

In vivo: In a live animal.

Metrorrhagia: Normal uterine bleeding at an abnormal time.

Mucilaginous: Substance that is slimy, gooey, sticky. It has the property of moistening, soothing, and helping heal skin and mucous membranes.

Mutagenic: Substance that has the property of being able to induce genetic mutation.

Narcotic: Substance that lessens pain by causing depression of the central nervous system. Derived from the Greek *narkotikos,* meaning "benumbing."

Neuralgia: Pain in and originating along nerve fibers.

Nutritive: Substance that is ingested and provides nutrition.

Plant: Any flora of the Earth.

Pruritus: Itching; an inflammation of the skin that produces itching.

Purgative: Substance that cleanses the bowels.

Rhinitis: Inflammation of the sinus membranes beginning in the mucous membranes of the nose (*rhino* means "nose").

Sedative: Substance that has a calming and quieting action on specific organs or systems: cardiac, nervous, cerebral, spinal, etc.

Soporific: Producing sleep.

Spasmolytic: Antispasmodic.

Stimulant: Substance that increases the action of a specific organ system and/or induces a sense of well-being.

Sudorific: Substance that produces sweat.

Tannins: Astringent compounds in plants that protect the plant from yeasts, being eaten, and bacterial decay.

Tincture: Usually a combination of an herb, alcohol, and water. Useful because of the preservative and extractive properties of alcohol on herbs.

Tonic: Substance taken to strengthen the body or a particular system of the body, generally in the treatment of chronic disease. Loosely, a tonic "tones" whatever system it affects.

Urinary antiseptic: Substance that is antiseptic to the urinary tract.

Uterine tonifier: Substance that has a strengthening activity on the tissues of the uterus.

Vaginitis: Inflammation of the vagina, from irritation or infection.

Weed: Derogatory term for a plant, similar to a racial epithet.

Wort: From the old English *wyrt,* meaning a root or plant. In herbalism, an herb, usually used as a combined term, e.g., St. John's wort, liverwort.

RESOURCES

Cryptolepsis

Nana Nkatiah, P.O. Box 22489, Seattle, WA 98122

Bulk herbs, seeds, and shiitake mushrooms

Blessed Herbs, 109 Barre Plains Road, Oakham, MA 01068 (800) 489-4372,
  (508) 882-3839

Trinity Herbs, P.O. Box 1001, Graton, CA 95444 (707) 824-2040,
  Fax (707) 824-2050

Horizon Seeds, P.O. Box 69, Williams, OR 97544 (541) 846-6704

Vitamin C

Wholesale Nutrition, P.O. Box 3345, Saratoga, CA 95070 (800) 325-2664,
  (408) 871-9519, www.nutri.com

SUGGESTED READING

Duke, James A. *The Green Pharmacy*, Emmaus, PA: Rodale, 1998.

Fox, Nicols. *Spoiled*. New York: Basic Books, 1998. (The best overview of the rise of resistant bacteria in our food supply.)

Green, James. *The Herbal Medicine Maker's Handbook*. Forestville, CA: Wildlife and Green Publications, 1990.

Green, Mindy, and Kathi Keville. *Aromatherapy: A Complete Guide to the Healing Art*. Watsonville, CA: Crossing Press, 1995.

Griggs, Barbara. *Green Pharmacy*. Rochester, VT: Healing Arts Press, 1997.

Hoffmann, David. *The New Holistic Herbal*. Rockport, MA: Element, 1992.

Lappé, Marc. *When Antibiotics Fail*. Berkeley, CA: North Atlantic Books, 1986. (The best overview of the subject and the only one that puts it in its proper ecological perspective.)

Levy, Stuart. *The Antibiotic Paradox*. New York: Plenum, 1992.

Preston, Richard. *The Hot Zone*. New York: Random House, 1997.

SELECTED BIBLIOGRAPHY

Antibiotic-Resistant Bacteria and Disease

"Across the USA." *USA Today*, December 28, 1998, page 8A. Listing for Washington, D.C.

American Association for the Advancement of Science, *Science*. August 21, 1992. (Entire volume focuses on antibiotic-resistant bacteria.)

Bayles, Fred. "CDC System Allows Officials to Track Dangerous Bacteria." *USA Today*, September 16, 1998, page 11A.

Begley, Sharon. "The End of Antibiotics." *Newsweek*, March 28, 1994.

Billing, Jennifer, and Paul Sherman. "Antimicrobrial Functions of Spices: Why Some Like It Hot." *The Quarterly Review of Biology*, March 1998.

Business Bulletin. "Disease Strikes the Pumpkin Patch." *Wall Street Journal*, September 24, 1998, page A1.

Bryan, L. E. *Bacterial Resistance and Susceptibility to Chemotherapeutic Agents*. Cambridge: Cambridge University Press, 1982.

Center for Science in the Public Interest, *Protecting the Crown Jewels of Medicine: A Strategic Plan to Preserve the Effectiveness of Antibiotics*. Washington, D.C.: Center for Science in the Public Interest, 1998.

Chase, Marilyn. "A Recent Batch of Food Poisonings Puts Public on Alert." *Wall Street Journal*, June 29, 1998, page B1.

Editorial. "Antibiotic Overkill Boosts Risks." *USA Today*, September 17, 1998, page 14A.

Fackelmann, Kathleen. "Eradication Efforts Fail to Stop STDs in Cities." *USA Today*, December 7, 1998, page D1.

Fisher, Jeffery. "Epidemics: The New Age of Disease." *Nutrition Science News*, August 1995.

———. *The Plague Makers*. New York: Simon and Schuster, 1994.

Fox, Nicols. *Spoiled: The Dangerous Truth about a Food Chain Gone Haywire*. New York: Basic Books, 1998.

Hospital Infection Control Practices Advisory Board. "Recommendations for Preventing the Spread of Vancomycin Resistance." *Infection Control and Hospital Epidemiology*. February 1995, pages 105–113.

Jarvis, William. "Preventing the Emergence of Multidrug-Resistant Microorganisms through Antimicrobial Use Controls: The Complexity of the Problem." *Infection Control and Hospital Epidemiology*. August 1996, pages 490–495.

Lappé Marc. *When Antibiotics Fail*. Berkeley, CA: North Atlantic Books, 1986.

Levy, Stuart. *The Antibiotic Paradox*. New York: Plenum, 1992.

Lifeline. "On the Anti-TB Front." *USA Today*, June 24, 1998, page D1.

Manasse, Henri. "Antibiotic Resistant Bacteria and How to Deal with Them" (Letter to the Editor). *USA Today*, September 28, 1998, page 16A.

Manning, Anita. "'Antibacterial' Soaps May Create New Problems." *USA Today*, September 22, 1998, page 6D.

———. "Cuban Doctor Imprisoned for Warning of a Dengue Fever Outbreak." *USA Today*, July 16, 1998.

———. "Vaccines Urged in Wake of Outbreak of Pneumonia." *USA Today*, June 25, 1998, page D1.

Mitsuhashi, S. *Drug Action and Drug Resistance in Bacteria*. Tokyo: University of Tokyo Press, 1971.

Nationline Column. "Bacteria Outbreak." *USA Today*, September 24, 1998, page 3A.

O'Donnell, Jayne. "Estimates of *E.coli* Cases Double." *USA Today*, December 7, 1998, page 1A.

Panlilio, Adelisa, et al. "Methicillin-Resistant *Staphylococcus aureus* in U.S. Hospitals; 1975–1991." *Infection Control and Hospital Epidemiology*, October 1992, pages 582–586.

Preston, Richard. *The Hot Zone*. New York: Random House, 1997.

Public Citizen. "Sausage Laws." *The Inlander*, July 8, 1998, page 4.

Rubin, Rita. "Unpasteurized Orange Juice is *E. coli* Culprit." *USA Today*, November 4, 1998, page D1.

Shell, Ellen Ruppel. "Resurgence of a Deadly Disease." *Atlantic Monthly*, August 1997, pages 45–60.

Spotts, Peter. "Controlling Bacteria on the Farm." *Christian Science Monito,r* June 25, 1998, page B6.

Sternberg, Steve. "On El Nino's Deadly Tail." *USA Today*, July 2, 1998, page D1.

———. "Sarah Lee Recalls Hot Dogs, Other Meats." *USA Today*, December 23, 1998, page 1A.

———. "Science, Legwork Combine to Catch Deadly Virus." *USA Today*, July 6, 1998, pages 6–8D.

Stolberg, Sheryl Gay. "Superbugs: The Bacteria Antibiotics Can't Kill." *The New York Times Magazine*, August 2, 1998.

Various authors. "Principles of Judicious Use of Antimicrobial Agents for Pediatric Upper Respiratory Tract Infections." *Pediatrics*, January 1998.

Note: All Abstracts are from the NAPRALERT Database.

ACACIA

Arvigo, Rosita, and Michael Balick. *Rainforest Remedies: One Hundred Healing Herbs of Belize*. Twin Lakes, WI: Lotus Press, 1993.

Avirutnant, W., and A. Pongpan. "The Antimicrobial Activity of Some Thai Flowers and Plants." *Mahidol Univ J Pharm Sci* 10(3):81–86, 1983. Abstract.

Caceres, A., O. Cano, B. Samayoa, and L. Aguilar. "Plants Used in Guatemala for the Treatment of Gastrointestinal Disorders. 1. Screening of 84 Plants Against Enterobacteria." *J Ethnopharmacol* 301:55–73, 1990. Abstract.

Chhabra, S., and F. Uiso. "Antibacterial Activity of Some Tanzanian Plants Used in Traditional Medicine." *Fitoterapia* 62(6):499–503, 1991. Abstract.

Ellingwood, Finley. *American Materia Medica, Therapeutics, and Pharmacognosy*. Cincinnati: Eclectic Publications, 1919.

Etkin, N. "Antimalarial Plants Used by Hausa in Northern Nigeria." *Trop Doctor* 27(1):12–16, 1997. Abstract.

Farouk, A., et al. "Antiomicrobial Activity of Certain Sudanese Plants Used in Folkloric Medicine. Screening for Antibacterial Activity (1)." *Fitoterapia* 54(1):3–7, 1983. Abstract.

Felter, Harvey, and John Uri Lloyd. *King's American Dispensatory*. Cincinnati: Eclectic Publications, 1895.

Gessler, M., et al. "Screening Tanzanian Medicinal Plants for Antimalarial Activity." *Acta Tropica* 56(1):65–77, 1994. Abstract.

Le Grand, A., et al. "Anti-Infectious Phytotherapies of the Tree-Savannah of Senegal (West Africa). 2. Antimicrobial Activity of 33 species." *J Ethnopharmacol* 22(1):25–31, 1988. Abstract.

Majupuria, Trilock Chandra, and D. P. Joshi. *Religious and Useful Plants of Nepal and India*. Lashkar (Gwalior), India: M. Gupta, Lalitpur Colony, 1989.

Moore, Michael. *Medicinal Plants of the Desert and Danyon West*. Sante Fe: Museum of New Mexico Press, 1989.

Nabi, Q., et al. "Antimicrobial Activity of *Acacia nilotica* (L.) Willd. ex del. var. nilotica (mimosaceae)." *J Ethnopharmacol* 37(1):77–9, 1992. Abstract.

Ray, R., and S. Majumdar. "Antimicrobial Activity of Some Indian Plants." *Econ Bot* 30:317–320, 1976. Abstract.

Sawhney, A., et al. "Studies on the Rationale of African Traditional Medicine. Part 2. Preliminary Screening of Medicinal Plants for Anti-Gonoccoci Activity." *Pak J Sci Ind Res* 21(5/6):189–192, 1978. Abstract.

Wassel, G., et al. "Phytochemical Examination and Biological Studies of *Acacia nilotica* L. Willd and *Acacia farnesiana* L. Willd Growing in Egypt." *Egypt J Pharm Sci* 33(1/2):327–340, 1992. Abstract.

Werbach, Melvyn, and Michael Murray. *Botanical Influences on Illness.* Tarzana, CA: Third Line Press, 1994. Lists multiple abstracts.

ALOE

Arvigo, Rosita, and Michael Balick. *Rainforest Remedies: One Hundred Healing Herbs of Belize.* Twin Lakes, WI: Lotus Press, 1993.

Chen, C., et al. "Development of Natural Crude Drug Resources from Taiwan (IV). In Vitro Studies of the Inhibitory Effect on 12 Microorganisms." *Shoyakugaku Zasshi* 41(3):215–225, 1987. Abstract.

Ellingwood, Finley. *American Materia Medica, Therapeutics, and Pharmacognosy.* Cincinnati: Eclectic Publications, 1919.

Felter, Harvey, and John Uri Lloyd. *King's American Dispensatory.* Cincinnati: Eclectic Publications, 1895.

Gottshall, R., et al. "The Occurrence of Antibacteial Substances Active against *Mycobacterium tuberculosis* in Seed Plants." *J Clin Invest* 28:920–923, 1949. Abstract.

Higgers, J., et al. "Dermaide Aloe/Aloe Vera Gel: Comparison of the Antimicrobial Effects." *J Am Med Technol* 41:293–294, 1979. Abstract.

Lorenzetti, L., et al. "Bacteriostatic Property of Aloe Vera." *J Pharm Sci* 53:1287, 1964. Abstract.

Suga, T., and T. Hirata. "The Efficacy of the Aloe Plant's Chemical Constituents and Biological Activities." *Cosmet Toiletries* 98(6):105–108, 1983. Abstract.

Werbach, Melvyn, and Michael Murray. *Botanical Influences on Illness.* Tarzana, CA: Third Line Press, 1994. Lists multiple abstracts.

CYPTOLEPSIS

Boye, G. L. "Antimalarial Action of *Cryptolepsis sanguinolenta* Extract." *The International Symposium on East-West Medicine,* chapter 14, pages 242–255, 1989.

Cimanga, K., et al. "In Vitro Activities of Alkaloids from *Cryptolepsis sanguinolenta.*" *Planta Medica* 62(1): 22–27, 1996. Abstract.

———. "In Vitro and Vivo Antiplasmodial Activity of Cryptolepene and Related Alkaloids from *Cryptolepsis sanguinolenta.*" *J Natural Products* 60(7): 688–691, 1997. Abstract.

Dean, Karen. "Cryptolepine Analogs" and "Cryptolepis." *HerbalGram,* no. 42, spring 1998, page 21.

Greller, P., et al. "Antimalarial Activity of Cryptolepine and Isocryptolepine, Alkaloids Isolated from *Cryptolepsis sanguinolenta.*" *Phytother Res* 10(4):317–321, 1996. Abstract.

Paulo, A., et al. "In Vitro Screening of *Cryptolepsis sanguinolenta* Alkaloids,." *J Ethnopharmacol* 44(2):127–130, 1994. Abstract.

ECHINACEA

Bergner, Paul. *The Healing Power of Echinacea and Goldenseal.* Rocklin, CA: Prima Publishing, 1997. Multiple trials and studies listed.

Blumenthal, Mark. "Echinacea Highlighted as Cold and Flu Remedy." *HerbalGram*, no. 29, spring/summer 1993, page 8.

Ellingwood, Finley. *American Materia Medica, Therapeutics, and Pharmacognosy.* Cincinnati: Eclectic Publications, 1919.

Felter, Harvey, and John Uri Lloyd. *King's American Dispensatory.* Cincinnati: Eclectic Publications, 1895.

Hobbs, Christopher. *The Echinacea Handbook.* Portland, OR: Eclectic Medical Publications, 1989. Multiple studies and trials listed.

McCaleb, Rob. "Echinacea Prevents Systemic *Candida* and *Listeria*." *HerbalGram*, no. 26, winter 1992, page 26.

Moore, Michael. *Medicinal Plants of the Desert and Danyon West.* Sante Fe: Museum of New Mexico Press, 1989.

Mowrey, Daniel. *The Scientific Validation of Herbal Medicine.* New Canaan, CT: Keats, 1986. Lists multiple abstracts of clinical trials and studies.

Weiss, Rudolph. *Herbal Medicine.* Sweden: Beaconsfield, 1988.

Werbach, Melvyn, and Michael Murray. *Botanical Influences on Illness.* Tarzana, CA: Third Line Press, 1994. Lists multiple abstracts of clinical trials and studies.

EUCALYPTUS

Alkofahi, A., et al. "Antimicrobial Evaluation of Some Plant Extracts of Traditional Medicine of Jordan." *Alex J Pharm Sci* 10(2):123–126, 1996. Abstract.

Aswal, B., et al. "Screening of Indian Plants for Biological Activity, Part X." *Indian J Exp Biol* 22(6):312–332, 1984. Abstract.

Badam, L., et al. "In Vitro Antimalarial Activity of Medicial Plants of India." *Indian J Med Res* 87(4):379–383, 1988. Abstract.

Barnabas, C., and S. Nagarajan. "Antimicrobial Activity of Flavionoids of Some Medicinal Plants." *Fitoterapia* 59(6):508–510, 1988. Abstract.

Begun, J., et al. "Studies of Essential Oils for Their Antibacterial and Antifungal Properties. Part 1. Preliminary Screening of 35 Essential Oils." *Bangladesh J Sci Ind Res* 28(4):25–34, 1993. Abstract.

Benouda, A., et al. "In Vitro Antibacterial Properties of Essential Oils, Tested against Hospital Pathogenic Bacteria." *Fitoterapia* 59(2):115–119, 1988. Abstract.

"Botanicals Containing Phytochemical Antagonists of Specific Micro-Organisms." *Protocol Journal of Botanical Medicine*, vol. 1, no. 1, summer 1995, pages 144–146.

Brantner, A., and E. Grein. "Antibacterial Activity of Plant Extracts Used Externally in Traditional Medicine." *J Ethnopharmacol*, 44(1):35–40, 1994. Abstract.

Chaudhari, D., and R. Suri. "Comparitive Studies on Chemical and Antimicrobial Activities of Fast Growing Eucalyptus Hybrid (fri-4 and fri-5) with Their Parents." *Indian Perfum* 35(1):30–34, 1991. Abstract.

Dellacassa, E., et al. "Antimicrobial Activity of Eucalyptus Essential Oils." *Fitoterapia* 60(6):544–546, 1989. Abstract.

Ellingwood, Finley. *American Materia Medica, Therapeutics, and Pharmacognosy.* Cincinnati: Eclectic Publications, 1919.

Felter, Harvey, and John Uri. *King's American Dispensatory.* Cincinnati: Eclectic Publications, 1895.

Hajji, F., et al. "Antimicrobial Activity of Twenty-one Eucalyptus Essential Oils." *Fitoterapia* 64(1):71–77, 1993. Abstract.

Hmamouchi, M., et al. "Report on the Antibacterial and Antifungal Properties of the Essential Oils of Eucalyptus." *Plant Med Phytother* 24(4):278–289, 1990. Abstract.

Ingram, Cass. *Killed on Contact: The Tea Tree Oil Story: Nature's Finest Antiseptic.* Cedar Rapids, IA: Literary Visions, 1992.

Janssen, A., et al. "Screening for Antimicrobial Activity of Some Essential Oils by the Agar Overlay Technique." *Pharm Weekbl (Sci Ed)* 8(6):289–292, 1986. Abstract.

McCaleb, Rob. "Tea Tree Oil and Antibiotic Resistant Bacteria." *HerbalGram*, no. 36, spring 1996, page 18.

Moore, Michael. *Medicinal Plants of the Desert and Danyon West.* Sante Fe: Museum of New Mexico Press, 1989.

Muanza, D., et al. "Antibacterial and Antifungal Activities of Nine Medicinal Plants from Zaire." *Int J Pharmacog* 32(4):337–345, 1994. Abstract.

Olsen, Cynthia. *Australian Tea Tree Oil Guide.* Pagosa Springs, CO: Kali Press, 1991.

Ontengco, D., et al. "Screening for the Antibacterial Activity of Essential Oils from Some Philippine Plants." *Acta Manilana* 43:19–23, 1995. Abstract.

Perez, C., Anesini, C., "In Vitro Antibacterial Activity of Argentine Folk Medicinal Plants Against *Salmonella typhi.*" *J Ethnopharmacol* 44(1):41–46, 1994. Abstract.

Prakash, S., et al. "Antibacterial and Antifungal Properties of Some Essential Oils Extracted from Medicinal Plants of the Kumaon Region." *Indian Oil Soap J* 37(9):230–232, 1972. Abstract.

Ross, S., et al. "Antimicrobial Activity of Some Egyptian Aromatic Plants." *Fitoterapia* 51:201–205, 1980. Abstract.

Saeed, M., and A. Sabir. "Antimicrobial Studies of the Constituents of Pakistani Eucalyptus Oils." *J Fac Pharm Gazi* 12(2):129–140, 1995. Abstract.

Suri, R., and T. Thind. "Antibacterial Activity of Some Essential Oils." *Indian Drugs Pharm Ind* 13:25–28, 1978. Abstract.

GARLIC

Abdullah, T. H., et al. "Garlic Revisited: Therapeutic for the Major Diseases of Our Time?" *J Nat Med Assoc* 80(4):439–445, 1988.

Ahsan, M., et al. "Garlic Extracts and Allicin: Broad Spectrum Antibacterial Agents Effective against Multiple Drug Resistant Strains of *Shigella dysenteriae* type 1 and *Shigella flexneri,* enterotoxigenic *Escherichia coli* and *Vibrio cholerae.*" *Phytother Res* 10(4):329–331, 1996. Abstract.

Anon. "Garlic in Cryptoccal Meningitis. A Preliminary Report of 21 Cases. *Chung-Hua I hsueh Tsa Chih (English Edition)* 93:123–126, 1980. Abstract.

Bergner, Paul. *The Healing Power of Garlic.* Rocklin, CA: Prima Publishing, 1996. Multiple abstracts and sources listed.

Block, Eric. "The Chemistry of Garlic and Onions." *Scientific American,* 252:114–119, 1985.

Chowdhury, A., et al. "Efficacy of Aqueous Extract of Garlic and Allicin in Experimental Shigellosis in Rabbits." *Indian J Med Res* [A] 93(1):33–36, 1991. Abstract.

Duke, James A. *The Green Pharmacy.* Emmaus, PA: Rodale, 1998.

Elnima, E., et al. "The Antimicrobial Activity of Garlic and Onion Extract." *Pharmazie* 38:747–748, 1983.

Foster, Steven. *Garlic.* Austin, TX:American Botanical Council, 1991.

Koch, Heinrich, and Larry Lawson. *Garlic: The Science and Therapeutic Application of Allium Sativum and Related Species.* Baltimore: Williams and Wilkins, 1996. The best overall look at hundreds of studies.

McCaleb, Rob. "The Latest in Garlic Research." *HerbalGram,* no. 30, winter 1994, page 11.

———. "Strong Association Between *Allium* Consumption and Cancer Protection." *HerbalGram,* no. 42, spring 1998, page 15.

Mintaraisit, A., et al. "Antibacterial Activity of Hom Daeng *(Allium ascalonisum L.).*" Abstract of 10th conference of science and technology, Thailand. Chiengmai, Thailand, 1984. Abstract.

Schmidt, M., et al. *Beyond Antibiotics.* Berkeley, CA: North Atlantic, 1994. Multiple studies listed.

Singh, K. V., and N. P. Shukla. 1984. "Activity on Multiple Resistant Bacteria of Garlic *(Allium sativum)* Extract." *Fitoterapia* 55(5):313–315, 1984.

Walker, Morton. *The Healing Powers of Garlic.* Stamford, CT: New Way of Life, 1988. Multiple studies listed.

GINGER

"Botanicals Containing Phytochemical Antagonists of Specific Micro-Organisms." *Protocol Journal of Botanical Medicine,* vol. 1, no. 1, summer 1995, pages 144–146.

Duke, James A. *The Green Pharmacy.* Emmaus, PA: Rodale, 1998.

Etkin, N. "Antimalarial Plants Used by Hausa in Northern Nigeria." *Trop Doctor* 27(1):12–16, 1997. Abstract.

Felter, Harvey, and John Uri Lloyd. *King's American Dispensatory.* Cincinnati: Eclectic Publications, 1895.

Fulder, Stephen. *The Ginger Book.* New York: Avery, 1996.

George, M., and K. Pandalai. "Investigations on Plant Antibiotics. Part IV. Further Research for Antibiotic Substances in Indian Medicinal Plants." *Indian J Med Res* 37:169–181, 1949. Abstract.

Janssen, A., and J. Scheffer. "Acetoxychavicol Acetate, an Antifungal Component of *Alpinia galanga.*" *Planta Med* 1985(6):507–511, 1985. Abstract.

Landis, Robyn, and K. P. Khalsa. *Herbal Defense.* New York: Warner Books, 1997.

Mascolo, N. "Ethnopharmacologic Investigation of Ginger *(Zingiber officinale).*" *J Ethnopharmacol* 27(1/2):129–140, 1989. Abstract.

McCaleb, Rob. "Fresh Ginger Juice in Treatment of Kitchen Burns." *HerbalGram,* no. 16, spring 1988, page 6, citing Cai Liang-Ping. *J New Chinese Med,* 2:22, 1984.

Misas, C., et al. "Contribution to the Biological Evaluation of Cuban Plants, II." *Rev Cub Med Trop* 31:13–19, 1979. Abstract.

Mowrey, Daniel. *The Scientific Validation of Herbal Medicine.* New Canaan, CT: Keats, 1986. Lists multiple abstracts of clinical trials.

Oloke, J., et al. "The Antibacterial and Antifungal Activities of Certain Components of *Aframomun melegueta* Fruits." *Fitoterapia* 59(5):384–388, 1988. Abstract.

Ontengco, D., et al. "Screening for the Antibacterial Activity of Essential Oils from Some Philippine Plants." *Acta Manilana* 43:19–23, 1995. Abstract.

Ray, R., and S. Majumdar. "Antimicrobial Activity of Some Indian Plants." *Econ Bot* 30:317–320, 1976. Abstract.

Ross, S., et al. "Antimicrobial Activity of Some Egyptian Aromatic Plants." *Fitoterapia* 51:201–205, 1980. Abstract.

Schmidt, M., et al. *Beyond Antibiotics.* Berkeley, CA: North Atlantic, 1994. Multiple studies listed.

Sinha, A., et al. "Antibacterial Study of Some Essential Oils." *Indian Perfum* 20:25–27, 1979. Abstract.

———. "Antimicrobial Properties of Essential Oils from *Zingiber chrysthanum* Leaves and Rhizomes." *Fitoterapia* 63(1):73–75, 1992. Abstract.

Weil, Andrew. *Eight Weeks to Optimum Health,* New York: Knopf, 1998.

Werbach, Melvyn, and Michael Murray. *Botanical Influences on Illness.* Tarzana, CA: Third Line Press, 1994. Lists multiple abstracts of clinical trials and studies.

GOLDENSEAL

Bergner, Paul. *The Healing Power of Echinacea and Goldenseal and Other Immune System Herbs.* Rocklin, CA: Prima Publishing, 1997.

Cech, Richo. "Comparison of a Few Goldenseal Analogues." Self-published, 1996.

Cech, R., et al. "The Presence of Significant Quantities of Berberine and Hydrastine in the Leaf and Stem of Organically Cultivated Goldenseal *(Hydrastis canadensis).*" Publication data not available, from a copy of the analysis, 1996.

D'Amico, M. "Investigation of the Presence of Substances Having Antibiotic Action in Higher Plants." *Fitoterapia* 21:77–82, 1950. Abstract.

Foster, Steven. *Goldenseal.* Botanical Series No. 309. Austin, TX: American Botanical Council, 1991.

Gottshall, R., et al. "The Occurrence of Antibacterial Substances Active Against *Mycobacterium tuberculosis* in Seed Plants." *J Clin Invest* 28:920–923, 1949. Abstract.

Gupte, S. "Use of Berberine in Treatment of Giardiasis." *Am J Dis Child* 129:866, 1975. Abstract.

Hartzell, A., and F. Wilcoxon. "A Survey of Plant Products for Insecticidal Properties." *Contr Boyce Thompson Inst* 12:127–141, 1941. Abstract.

Kaneyda, Y., et al. "In Vitro Effects of Berberine Sulphate on the Growth and Structure of *Entamorba histolytica, Giardia lamblia,* and *Trichomonas vaginalis.*" *Ann Tropical Med Parasitol* 85(4):417–425, 1991. Abstract.

Maung, U., et al. "Clinical Trial of Berberine in Acute Watery Diarrhea." *Br Med J,* 291(7):1601–1605, 1985. Abstract.

Mowrey, Daniel. *The Scientific Validation of Herbal Medicine.* New Canaan, CT: Keats, 1986. Lists multiple abstracts of clinical trials, primarily on berberine.

Rabbani, G. H., et al. "Randomized Controlled Trial of Berberine Sulphate Therapy for Diarrhea Due to Enterotoxigenic *Escherichia coli* and *Vibrio cholerae.*" *J Infect Dis,* 155(5):979–984, 1985.

Sack, R., et al. "Berberine Inhibits Intestinal Secretory Response of *Vibrio cholerae* and *Escherichia coli* enterotoxins." *Infection Immunity* 35(2):471–475, 1982. Abstract.

Snow, Joanne Marie. "*Hydrastis canadensis* L. (Ranunculaceae)." *Protocol Journal of Botanical Medicine,* vol. 2, no. 2, 1997. Lists multiple abstracts of clinical trials and laboratory studies mostly on berberine.

Werbach, Melvyn, and Michael Murray. *Botanical Influences on Illness*. Tarzana, CA: Third Line Press, 1994. Lists multiple abstracts of clinical trials, primarily on berberine.

GRAPEFRUIT SEED EXTRACT

Caceres, A., et al. "Screening of Antimicrobial Activity of Plants Popularly Used in Guatemala for the Treatment of Dermatomucosal Diseases." *J Ethnopharmacol* 20(3):223–237, 1987. Abstract.

Chen, C., et al. "Development of Natural Crude Drug Resources from Taiwan (IV). In Vitro Studies of the Inhibitory Effect on 12 Microorganisms." *Shoyakugaku Zasshi* 41(3):215–225, 1987. Abstract.

Ebana, R., et al. "Microbiological Exploitation of Cardiac Glycosides and Alkaloids from *Garcinia kola, Borreria ocymoides, Kola nitida*, and *Citrus aurantifolia*." *J Appl Bacteriol* 71(5):398–401, 1991. Abstract.

Hussain, H., and Y. Deeni. "Plants in Kano Ethnomedicine: Screening for Antimicrobial Activity and Alkaloids." *Int J Pharmacog* 29(1):51–56, 1991. Abstract.

Misas, C., et al. "Contribution to the Biological Evaluation of Cuban Plants." *Rev Cub Med Trop* 31:37–43, 1979. Abstract.

Perez, C., and C. Anesini. "In Vitro Antibacterial Activity of Argentine Folk Medicinal Plants against *Salmonella typhi*." *J Ethnopharmacol* 44 1:41–46, 1994. Abstract.

Ross, S., et al. "Antimicrobial Activity of Some Egyptian Aromatic Plants." *Fitoterapia* 51:201–205, 1980. Abstract.

Sharamon, Shalila, and Bodo Baginski. *The Healing Power of Grapefruit Seed*. Twin Lakes, WI: Lotus Light, 1997. Cites 140 research papers, laboratory studies, and *in vivo, in vitro*, and human trials. Though the book itself is weak in some areas, it is the best overall source for research done on grapefruit seed extract.

Uhlenbrock, S. "Grapefruit Seed Extract: Naturally Good for All?" *Pharmazie* 141 (42):46–48, 1996. Abstract.

Werbach, Melvyn, and Michael Murray. *Botanical Influences on Illness*. Tarzana, CA: Third Line Press, 1994. Lists multiple abstracts of clinical trials and studies.

HONEY

Aasved, Mikal. *Alcohol, Drinking and Intoxication in Preindustrial Society: Theoretical, Nutritional, and Religious Considerations*. Ph.D. dissertation, University of California, Santa Barbara, 1988.

al Somal, N., et al. *J R Soc Med*, 87(1): 9, 1994, and Postmes, T. et al. *Lancet* 341: 756, 1993 [see also 341:90, 1993] cited in Patrick Quillin, *Honey, Garlic, and Vinegar*. North Canton, OH: The Leader Company, 1996.

Ali, A. T., and M. N. Chowdhury, et al. "Inhibitory Effect of Natural Honey on *Helicobacter pylori*." *Trop Gastroenterol* 12(3):139–143, 1991 cited in Elkins, *Bee Pollen*.

Beck, Bodog, and Doree Smedley. *Honey and Your Health*. New York:Robert McBride, 1944, page 35.

Brown, Royden. *Royden Brown's Bee Hive Product Bible*. Garden City, NY: Avery Publishing, 1993.

Dustmann, J.H. "Bee Products for Human Health." *American Bee Journal*, vol. 136, no. 4, 1996, page 275.

Elbagoury, E. F., and S. Rasmy. "Antibacterial Action of Natural Honey on Anaerobic Bacteroides" *J Egypt Dent* 39(1):381–86, 1993, and Ndayisaba, G., L. Bazira, and E. Haboniman. "Treatment of Wounds with Honey." *Presse-Med* 21(32):1516–8, 1992, cited in Elkins, *Bee Pollen*.

Elkins, Rita. *Bee Pollen, Royal Jelly, Propolis, and Honey*. Pleasant Grove, UT: Woodland Publishing, 1996.

Harmon, Ann. "Hive Products for Therapeutic Use." *American Bee Journal*, vol. 123, no. 1, 1983.

Kotova, Galina. "Apiary Products Are Important in Soviet Medicine." *American Bee Journal*, vol. 121, no. 12, 1981, page 850.

Krochmal, Connie and Arnold. "Apitherapy in Romania." *American Bee Journal*, vol. 121, no. 11, 1981, page 786.

Phuapradit, W. et al., *Aust N Z J Obstet Gynecol* 32(4):381, 1992, and Efem, S.E., *Surgery* 113(2):200, 1993, cited in ibid.

Postumes, T., E. van den Bogaard, and M. Hazen. "Honey for Wounds, Ulcers, and Skin Graft Preservation." *Lancet* 341:756–757, 1993, cited in Root-Bernstein, *Honey, Mud, and Maggots*.

Quillin, Patrick. *Honey, Garlic, and Vinegar*. North Canton, OH: The Leader Company, 1996.

Root-Bernstein, Robert and Michele. *Honey, Mud, and Maggots*, Boston: Houghton Mifflin, 1997.

Schmidt, Justin. "Apitherapy Meeting Held in the Land of Milk and Honey." *American Bee Journal*, vol. 136, no. 10, 1996, page 722.

Subrahmanyam, M. *B J Plast Surg* 46(4):322, 1993, cited in Quillin, *Honey, Garlic, and Vinegar*.

JUNIPER

Bagci, E., and M. Digrak. "Antimicrobial Activity of Essential Oils of Some Abies (fir) Species from Turkey." *Flavour Fragrance J* 11(4):251–256, 1996. Abstract.

Bhakuni, D., et al. "Screening of Indian Plants for Biological Activity, Part III." *Indian J Exp Biol* 9:91, 1971. Abstract.

Bonsignore, L., et al. "A Preliminary Screening of Sardinian Plants." *Fitoterapia* 61(4):339–341, 1990. Abstract.

"Botanicals Containing Phytochemical Antagonists of Specific Micro-Organisms." *The Protocol Journal of Botanical Medicine*, vol. 1 no. 1, 1995, pages 144–146.

Buhner, Stephen Harrod. *Sacred and Herbal Healing Beers*. Boulder, CO: Siris, 1998.

Clark, A., et al. "Antimicrobial Properties of Heartwood, Bark/Sapwood and Leaves of *Juniperus* Species." *Phytother Res* 4(1):15–19, 1990. Abstract.

Dye, Michael. "Our Health, Disease, and 'Old Age' Are Formed on the Molecular Battlefield of Antioxidents vs. Free Radicals." *Back to the Garden*, Winter 1994/95.

Ellingwood, Finley. *American Materia Medica, Therapeutics, and Pharmacognosy*. Cincinnati: Eclectic Publications, 1919.

Felter, Harvey, and John Uri Lloyd. *King's American Dispensatory*. Cincinnati: Eclectic Publications, 1895.

Janssen, A., et al. "Screening for Antimicrobial Activity of Some Essential Oils by the Agar Overlay Technique." *Pharm Weekbl (Sci Ed)* 8(6):289–292, 1986. Abstract.

Kartning, T., et al. "Antimicrobial Activity of the Essential Oil of Young Pine Shoots *(Picea abies L.)*." *J Ethnopharmacol* 35(2):155–157, 1991. Abstract.

Kindra, K., and T. Satyanarayana. "Inhibitory Activity of Essential Oils of Some Plants against Pathogenic Bacteria." *Indian Drugs* 16:15–17, 1978. Abstract.

McChesney, J., and R. Adams. "Co-evaluation of Plant Extracts as Petrochemical Substitutes and for Biologically Active Compounds." *Econ Bot* 39(1):74–86, 1985. Abstract.

Mishra, P., and C. Chauhan. "Antimicrobial Studies of the Essential Oil of the Berries of *Juniperus macropoda* Boiss." *Hindustan Antibiotics* 26(1/2):38–40, 1984. Abstract.

Moore, Michael. *Medicinal Plants of the Mountain West.* Sante Fe: Museum of New Mexico Press, 1979.

Mowrey, Daniel. *The Scientific Validation of Herbal Medicine.* New Canaan, CT: Keats, 1986. Lists multiple abstracts of clinical trials, primarily on berberine.

Muhammad, I., et al. "Antibacterial Diterpenes from the Leaves and Seeds of *Juniperus excelsa* M. Bieb." *Phytother Res* 6(5):261–264, 1992. Abstract.

Paterson, Andrew. *Protection for Life.* Crystal Clear Publications, 1995.

Recio, M., et al. "Antimicrobial Activity of Selected Plants Employed in the Spanish Mediterranean Area, Part II." *Phytother Res* 3(3):77–80, 1989. Abstract.

Richardson, M., et al. "Bioactivity Screening of Plants Selected on the Basis of Folkloric Use or Presence of Lignans in a Family." *Phytother Res* 6:274–278 , 1992. Abstract.

LICORICE

Acharya, S., et al. "A Preliminary Open Trial on Interferon Stimulator Derived from *Glycyrrhiza glabra* in the Treatment of Subacute Hepatic Failure." *Indian J Med Res* 98(2):69–74, 1993. Abstract.

Al-shamma, A., and Mitscher, L. "Comprehensive Survey of Indigenous Iraqi Plants for Potential Economic Value. I. Screening Results of 327 Species for Alkaloids and Antimicrobial Agents." *J Nat Prod* 42:633–642, 1979.

Bannister, B. "Cardiac Arrest Due to Liquorice-Induced Hypokalemia." *Br Med J* 1977(2):738, 1977.

"Botanicals Containing Phytochemical Antagonists of Specific Micro-Organisms." *Protocol Journal of Botanical Medicine,* 1(1):144–146, 1995.

Ellingwood, Finley. *American Materia Medica, Therapeutics, and Pharmacognosy.* Cincinnati: Eclectic Publications, 1919.

Felter, Harvey, and John Uri Lloyd. *King's American Dispensatory.* Cincinnati: Eclectic Publications, 1895.

Fitzpatrick, F. "Plant Substances Active against *Mycobacterium tuberculosis*." *Antibiot Chemother* 4:528, 1954. Abstract.

Hrelia, P., et al. "Potential Antimutagenic Activity of *Glycyrrhiza glabra* extract." *Phytother Res* 10:S101–S103, 1996. Abstract.

Leslie, G. "A Pharmacometric Evaluation of Nine Bio-Strath Herbal Remedies." *Medita* 8(10):3–19, 1978. Abstract.

Mira, P., et al. "Antimalarial Activity of Traditional Plants against Erythrocytic Stages of *Plasmodium berghei*." *Int J Pharmacog* 29(1):19–23, 1991. Abstract.

Mitscher, L., et al. "Antimicrobial Agents from Higher Plants. Antimicrobial Isoflavionoids and Related Substances from *Glycyrhiza glabra* L. var. typica." *J Nat Prod* 43:259–269, 1980. Abstract.

———. "Antimicrobial Agents from Higher Plants, *Glycyrrhiza glabra* (var. Spanish): I. Some Antimicrobial Isoflavans, Isoflavenes, Flavones, and Isoflavones. *Heterocycles* 9:1533, 1978. Abstract.

Moore, Michael. *Medicinal Plants of the Mountain West.* Sante Fe: Museum of New Mexico Press, 1979.

Namba, T., et al. "Studies on Dental Caries Prevention by Traditional Medicines, Part VII. Screening of Ayurevedic Medicines for Anti-Plaque Action." *Shoyakugaku Zasshi* 39(2):146–153, 1985. Abstract.

Ngo, H., et al. "Modulation of Mutagenesis, DNA Binding, and Metabolism of Aflatoxin B1 by Licorice Compounds." *Nut Res* 12(2):247–257, 1992. Abstract.

Okada, K., et al. "Identification of Antimicrobial and Antioxident Constituents from Licorice of Russian and Xinjiang Origin." *Chem Pharm Bull* 37(9):2528–2530, 1989. Abstract.

Ray, P., and S. Majumdar. "Antimicrobial Activity of Some Indian Plants." *Econ Bot* 30:317–320, 1976. Abstract.

Shirinyan, E., et al. "9,11,13-Trihydroxy-10(E)-Ocadecenic and 9,12,13-Trihydroxy-10,11-Epoxoctadecaonic Acids. New Antistressor Compounds from Liquorice." *IZV Akad Nauk SSR* 1988(6):932–936, 1988. Abstract.

Sigurjonsdottir, H., et al. "Is Blood Pressure Commonly Raised by Moderate Consumption of Liquorice?" *J Human Hypertension* 9(5):345–348, 1995. Abstract.

Snow, Joanne. "*Glycyrrhiza glabra.*" *Protocol Journal of Botanical Medicine* 1(3):9–14, Winter 1996.

Taylor, A., and F. Bartter. "Hypertension in Licorice Intoxication, Acromegaly, and Cushing's Syndrome." *Hypertens Physiopathol Treat* 1977:755, 1977. Abstract.

Watanabe, S., et al. "Release of Secretin of Liquorice Extract in Dogs." *Pancreas* 1(5):449–454, 1986. Abstract.

SAGE

Alkofahi, A., et al. "Antimicrobial Evaluation of Some Plant Extracts of Traditional Medicine of Jordan." *Alex J Pharm Sci* 10(2):123–126, 1996 Abstract.

Ahmed, S., et al. "Antibacterial Activity of *Salvia santolinifolia.*" *Fitoterapia* 65(3):271–272, 1994. Abstract.

Alkofahi, A., et al. "Antimicrobial Evaluation of Some Plant Extracts of Traditional Medicine of Jordan." *Alex J Pharm Sci* 10(2):123–126, 1996 Abstract.

Anesini, C., and C. Perez. "Screening of Plants Used in Argentine Folk Medicine for Antimicrobrial Activity." *J Ethnopharmacol* 39(2):119–128, 1993. Abstract.

"Botanicals Containing Phytochemical Antagonists of Specific Micro-Organisms." *Protocol Journal of Botanical Medicine.* 1(1):144–146, 1995.

Brantner, A., and E. Grein. "Antibacterial Activity of Plant Extracts Used Externally in Traditional Medicine." *J Ethnopharmacol,* 44(1):35–40, 1994. Abstract.

Derbentseva, N., et al. "Antimicrobial Substances from Garden Sage (*Salvia officinalis* L.)" *Mikrobiol Zhur* 21(6):43–47, 1959. Abstract.

Duke, James A. *The Green Pharmacy.* Emmaus, PA: Rodale Press, 1998.

El-keltawi, N., et al. "Antimicrobial Activity of Some Egyptian Aromatic Plants." *Herba Pol* 26(4):245–250, 1980. Abstract.

Ellingwood, Finley. *American Materia Medica, Therapeutics, and Pharmacognosy.* Cincinnati: Eclectic Publications, 1919.

Felter, Harvey, and John Uri Lloyd. *King's American Dispensatory.* Cincinnati: Eclectic Publications, 1895.

Gottshall, R., et al. "The Occurrence of Antibacteial Substances Active against *Mycobacterium tuberculosis* in Seed Plants." *J Clin Invest* 28:920–923, 1949. Abstract.

Jalsenjak, V., et al. "Microcapsules of Sage Oil: Essential Oils Content and Antimicrobial Activity." *Pharmazie* 42(6):419–420, 1987. Abstract.

Janssen, A., et al. "Screening for Antimicrobial Activity of Some Essential Oils by the Agar Overlay Technique" *Pharm Weekbl (Sci Ed)* 8(6):289–292, 1986. Abstract.

Leslie, G. "A Pharmacometric Evaluation of Nine Bio-Strath Herbal Remedies." *Medita* 8(10):3–19, 1978. Abstract.

Moore, Michael. *Medicinal Plants of the Mountain West.* Sante Fe: Museum of New Mexico Press, 1979.

Nadir, M. "The Effect of Different Methods of Extraction on the Antimicrobial Activity of Medicinal Plants" *Fitoterapia* 57(5):355–364, 1986. Abstract.

Recio, M., et al. "Antimicrobial Activity of Selected Plants Employed in the Spanish Mediterranean Area, Part II." *Phytother Res* 3(3):77–80, 1989. Abstract.

Ross, S., et al. "Antimicrobial Activity of Some Egyptian Aromatic Plants." *Fitoterapia* 51:201–205, 1980. Abstract.

Sabri, N., et al. "Two New Rearranged Abietane Dipertene Quinones from *Salvia aegyptiaca* L." *J Org Chem* 54(17):4097–4099, 1989. Abstract.

Shabana, M., et al. "Study of Wild Egyptian Plants of Potential Medicinal Activity Sixth Communication: Antibacterial and Antifungal Activities of Some Selected Plants." *Arch Exp Veterinaermed* 42(5):737–741, 1988. Abstract.

Sivropoulou, A., et al. "Antimicrobial, Cytotoxic, and Antiviral Activities of *Salvia fructiosa* Essential Oil." *J Agr Food Chem* 45(8):3197–3201, 1997. Abstract.

USNEA

Ahmadjian, V., and M. Hale. *The Lichens.* London: Academic Press, 1973, pages 547–713.

Al-Meshal, I., et al. "Phytochemical and Biological Screening of Saudi Medicinal Plants, Part I." *Fitoterapia* 53:79–84, 1982. Abstract.

Buhner, Stephen Harrod. *Sacred Plant Medicine.* Niwot, CO: Roberts Rinehart, 1996.

Hale, Mason. *The Biology of Lichens.* New York: American Elsevier Publishing Company, 1974.

Hobbs, Christopher. *Usnea: The Herbal Antibiotic.* Capitola, CA: Botanica Press, 1990.

Rowe, J., et al. "Antibacterial Activity of South Spain Lichens." *Ann Pharm Fr* 47 (2):89–94, 1989. Abstract.

———. "New Study of Antimicrobrial Activity and Identification of Lichenical Substances of Some Lichens From South Spain." *Ann Pharm Fr* 49(5):278–285, 1991. Abstract.

WORMWOOD

Acevedo, J., et al. "In Vitro Antimicrobrial Activity of Various Plant Extracts Used by Purepecha against Some Enterobacteriaceae." *Int J Pharmacognosy* 31(1):61–64, 1993. Abstract.

Akbar, S. "Anti-Hepatoxic Activity of *Salvia haematodes* (Wall.) and *Artemesia absinthium* (Linn.)." *IRCS Med Sci* 14:439–440, 1986. Abstract.

Al-Yahya, M., et al. "Phytochemical and Biological Screening of Saudi Medicinal Plants, Part II." *Fitoterapia* 54(1):21–24, 1983. Abstract.

Anesini, C., and C. Perez. "Inhibition of *Pseudomonas aerguinosa* by Argentinean Medicinal Plants." *Fitoterapia* 65(2):169–172, 1994. Abstract.

———. "Screening of Plants Used in Argentine Folk Medicine for Antimicrobial Activity." *J Ethnopharmacol* 39(2):119–128, 1993. Abstract.

Caceres, A., et al. "Plants Used in Guatemala for the Treatment of Dermatophytic Infections. 1. Screening for Antimycotic Activity of 44 Plant Extracts." *J Ethnopharmacol* 31(3):263–276, 1991. Abstract.

———. "Plants Used in Guatemala for the Treatment of Gastrointestinal Disorders. 1. Screening of 84 Plants Against Enterobacteria." *J Ethnopharmacol* 30(1):55–73, 1990. Abstract.

———. "Screening of Antimicrobial Activity of Plants Popularly Used in Guatemala for the Treatment of Dermatomucosal Diseases." *J Ethnopharmacol* 20(3):223–237, 1987. Abstract.

Carron, R., et al. "Antimicrobial Properties of Different Extracts Obtained from Some Mediterranean Plants of Medicinal Interest." *Plant Med Phytother* 21(4):195–202, 1987. Abstract.

Chen, C., et al. "Development of Natural Crude Drug Resources from Taiwan (VI). In Vitro Studies of the Inhibitory Effect on 12 Microorganisms." *Shoyakugaku Zasshi* 41(3):215–225, 1987. Abstract.

Chopra, C., et al. "In Vitro Antibacterial Activity of Oils from Indian Medicinal Plants." *J Am Pharm Assoc Sci Ed* 49:780, 1960. Abstract.

Demidov, V. "Biological Antiseptics in Certain Plants." *Bor'ba Potery v Zhivotnovodstve* 1963:183–200, 1963. Abstract.

Dopp, W., and H. Bersch. "Tuberculostatic Action of Some Plant Extracts in Vitro." *Pharmazie* 5:603–604, 1950. Abstract.

Ellingwood, Finley. *American Materia Medica, Therapeutics, and Pharmacognosy.* Cincinnati: Eclectic Publications, 1919.

Felter, Harvey, and John Uri Lloyd. *King's American Dispensatory.* Cincinnati: Eclectic Publications, 1895.

Francois, G., et al. "Antiplasmodial Activities of Sesquiterpent Lactones and Other Compounds in Organic Extracts of *Artemesia annua.*" *Planta Medica Suppl* 59 (7):A677–A678, 1993. Abstract.

George, M., and Pandalai, K. "Investigations on Plant Antibiotics. Part IV. Further Research for Antibiotic Substances in Indian Medicinal Plants." *Indian J Med Res* 37:169–181, 1949. Abstract.

Gilani, A., and K. Janbaz. "Preventative and Curative Effects of *Artemesia absinthium* on Acetaminophen and CCL4-Induced Hepatotoxicity." *Gen Pharmacol* 26(2):309–315, 1995. Abstract.

Grange, J., and R. Davey. "Detection of Antituberculosis Activity in Plant Extracts." *J Appl Bacteriol* 68(6):587–591, 1990. Abstract.

Han, B., et al. "Screening on the Anti-Inflammatory Activity of Crude Drugs." *Korean Journal of Pharmacognosy* 4(3):205–209, 1972. Abstract.

Hernandez, H., et al. "Effect of Aqueous Extracts of Artemesia on the In Vitro Culture of *Plasmodium falciparum.*" *Fitoterapia* 61(6):540–541, 1990. Abstract.

Janssen, A., et al. "Screening for Antimicrobial Activity of Some Essential Oils by the Agar Overlay Technique." *Pharm Weekbl (Sci Ed)* 8(6):289–292, 1986. Abstract.

Kaul, V., et al. "Antimicrobial Activities of the Essential Oils of *Artemesia absinthium*, *Artemesia vestita*, and *Artemesia vulgaris*." *Indian Journal of Pharmacy* 38:21, 1976. Abstract.

Khattak, S., et al. "Antipyretic Studies on Some Indigenous Pakistani Medicinal Plants." *J Ethnopharmacol* 14(1):45–51, 1985. Abstract.

Li, P. "Fumigation with *Artemesia vulgaris* Leaf for Inhibition of Bacterial Activity: Its Therapeutic Effects on Burns." *Chinese J Surg* 13:787, 1965. Abstract.

McCaleb, Rob. "Immunomodulating Compounds from Chinese Herbs." *HerbalGram*, no. 41, fall 1997, page 19.

McCaleb, Rob. "The Whole is Better." *HerbalGram*, no. 29, spring/summer 1993, page 20, citing Liu, K., et al. "Antimalarial Activity of *Artemisia annua* Flavionoids from Whole Plants and Cell Cultures. [Coll. Med., Natl. Taiwan Univ., Taipei, Taiwan] *Plant Cell Rep* 11(12):637–640.

Mendiola, J., et al. "Extracts of *Artemesia abrotanum* and *Artemesia absinthium* inhibit growth of *Naegleria flowleri* in vitro." *Trans R Soc Trop Med Hyg* 85(1):78–79, 1991. Abstract.

Moore, Michael. *Medicinal Plants of the Desert and Canyon West*. Sante Fe: Museum of New Mexico Press, 1989.

Perez, C., and C. Anesini. "In Vitro Antibacterial Activity of Argentine Folk Medicinal Plants Against *Salmonella typhii*." *J Ethnopharmacol* 44(1): 41–46, 1994. Abstract.

Recio, M., et al. "Antimicrobial Activity of Selected Plants Employed in the Spanish Mediterranean Area, Part II." *Phytother Res* 3(3):77–80, 1989. Abstract.

Shabana, M., et al. "Study of Wild Egyptian Plants of Potential Medicinal Activity Sixth Communication: Antibacterial and Antifungal Activities of Some Selected Plants." *Arch Exp Veterinaermed* 42(5):737–741, 1988. Abstract.

Van Hensbroek, M., et al. "A Trial of Artemether or Quinine in Children with Cerebral Malaria." *N Engl J Med* 335(2):69–75, 1996, and Hien, T. T., N. P. J. Day, N. H. Phu, *N Engl J Med* 335(2):76–83.

Weisbord, S., et al. "Poison On Line — Acute Renal Failure Caused by Oil of Wormwood Purchased Through the Internet." *N Engl J Med* 337 (12):825–827, 1997. Abstract.

Yashphe, J., et al. "Antibacterial Activity of *Artemesia herba-alba*." *J Pharm Sci* 68:924–925, 1979. Abstract.

Zafar, M. et al. "Screening of *Artemesia absinthium* for Antimalarial Effects on *Plasmodium berghei* in Mice: A Preliminary Report." *J Ethnopharmacol* 30(2):223–226, 1990. Abstract.

ASHWAGANDHA

Al-Meshal, I., et al. "Phytochemical and Biological Screening of Saudi Medicinal Plants, Part I." *Fitoterapia* 53:79–84, 1982. Abstract.

Boily, Y. "Screening of Medicinal Plants of Rwanda (Central Africa) for Antimicrobial Activity." *J Ethnopharmacol* 16(1):1–13, 1986. Abstract.

"Botanicals Containing Phytochemical Antagonists of Specific Micro-Organisms." *Protocol Journal of Botanical Medicine*, Vol. 1, No. 1, 1995, pages 144–146.

Farouk, A. "Antimicrobial Activity of Certain Sudanese Plants Used in Folkloric Medicine. Screening for Antimicrobial Activity." *Fitoterapia* 54(1):3–7, 1983. Abstract.

Felter, Harvey, and John Uri Lloyd. *King's American Dispensatory*. Cincinnati: Eclectic Publications, 1895.

Gaind, K., and R, Budhiraja. "Antibacterial and Anthelmintic Activity of *Withania coagulans.*" *Indian J Pharmacy* 29(6):185–186, 1967. Abstract.

Jaffer, H., et al. "Evaluation of Antimicrobial Activity of *Withania somnifera* Extracts." *Fitoterapia* 59(6):497–500, 1988. Abstract.

Khan, M., et al. "Antibacterial Activity of *Withania coagulans.*" *Fitoterapia* 64(4):367–370, 1993. Abstract.

Landis, Robyn, and K. P. Khalsa. *Herbal Defense.* New York: Warner Books, 1997.

Ray, R., and S. Majumdar. "Antimicrobial Activity of Some Indian Plants." *Econ Bot* 30:317–320, 1976. Abstract.

Weil, Andrew. *Eight Weeks to Optimum Health.* New York: Alfred A. Knopf, 1998.

Werbach, Melvyn, and Michael Murray. *Botanical Influences on Illness.* Tarzana, CA: Third Line Press, 1994. Multiple abstract listings.

ASTRAGALUS

"Botanicals Containing Phytochemical Antagonists of Specific Micro-Organisms." *Protocol Journal of Botanical Medicine,* vol. 1, no. 1, summer 1995, pages 144–146.

Choe, T. "Antibacterial Activities of Some Herb Drugs." *Korean J Pharmacog* 17(4):302–307, 1986. Abstract.

Gagnon, Daniel. "Seven Top Cold and Flu-Fighting Herbs." *Prevention,* December 1998.

Landis, Robyn, and K. P. Khalsa. *Herbal Defense.* Warner Books, 1997.

McCaleb, Rob. "Astragalus and Viral Heart Disease." *HerbalGram,* no. 24, winter 1991, page 20, citing Jiang and Xiao, *Handbook of Planta Medica.,* Beijing: People's Health Publishers, 1986, pages 127–128.

———. "Astragalus Enhances Natural Killer Cell Activity." *HerbalGram,* no. 21, fall 1989, page 16, citing *J Clin Lab Immunol* 25:112–123, 1988.

———. "Astragalus for the Liver." *HerbalGram,* no. 25, summer 1991, page 19, citing Yang, Y. Z., et al., *Chinese Med J* 107(7):595, 1987.

———. "Immune System Stimulation from Astragalus." *HerbalGram,* no. 17, summer 1988, page 24, citing *Cancer Research* 48:1410–5, 1988.

Ross, S., et al. "Studies for Determining Antibiotic Substances in Some Egyptian Plants. Part I. Screening for Antimicrobial Activity." *Fitoterapia* 51:303–308, 1980. Abstract.

Werbach, Melvyn, and Michael Murray. *Botanical Influences on Illness.* Tarzana, CA: Third Line Press, 1994. Multiple abstract listings.

Zolotnitskaya, S., et al. "The Antimicrobial Activity of Some Alkaloid-Containing Plants of the Armenian Flora" *IZV Akad Nauk Arm SSr Biol Nauki* 15(8):33, 1962. Abstract.

BONESET

Bergner, Paul. *The Healing Power of Echinacea and Goldenseal.* Rocklin, CA: Prima Publishing, 1997.

Boyd, L. "Pharmacology of the Homeopathic Drugs." *J Am Inst Homeopathy* 21:209, 1928. Abstract.

Ellingwood, Finley. *American Materia Medica, Therapeutics, and Pharmacognosy.* Cincinnati: Eclectic Publications, 1919.

Felter, Harvey, and John Uri Lloyd. *King's American Dispensatory.* Cincinnati: Eclectic Publications, 1895.

Gassinger, C., et al. "A Controlled Clinical Trial for Testing the Efficacy of the Homeopathic Drug *Eupatorium perfoliatum* D2 in the Treatment of Common Cold." *Arzneim-Forsch* 31:732–736, 1981. Abstract.

Moerman, Daniel. *Medicinal Plants of Native America.* Ann Arbor, MI: University of Michigan, Museum of Anthropology, Technical Reports, No. 19, 1986.

Muni, I., et al. "Cytoxicity of North Dakota Plants: I. In Vitro Studies." *J Pharm Sci* 56:50–54, 1967. Abstract.

Vollmar, A., et al. "Immunologically Active Polysaccharides of *Eupatorium cannabinum* and *Eupatorium perfoliatum.*" *Phytochemistry* 25(2):377–381, 1986. Abstract.

Wagner, H., et al. "Immunostimulating Polysaccharides of Higher Plants." *Arzneim-Forsch* 35(7):1069–1075, 1985. Abstract.

———. "Immunostimulating Polysaccharides of Higher Plants/Preliminary Communication." *Arzneim-Forsch* 34(6):659–661, 1984. Abstract.

Weiss, Rudolph. *Herbal Medicine.* Beaconsfield, England: Beaconsfield Pub. Ltd., 1988.

Wood, Matthew. *The Book of Herbal Wisdom."* Berkeley, CA: North Atlantic Books, 1998.

RED ROOT

Ellingwood, Finley. *American Materia Medica, Therapeutics, and Pharmacognosy.* Cincinnati: Eclectic Publications, 1919.

Felter, Harvey, and John Uri Lloyd. *King's American Dispensatory.* Cincinnati: Eclectic Publications, 1895.

Moerman, Daniel. *Medicinal Plants of Native America.* Ann Arbor, MI: University of Michigan, Museum of Anthropology, Technical Reports, No. 19, 1986.

Moore, Michael. *Medicinal Plants of the Mountain West.* Sante Fe: Museum of New Mexico Press, 1979.

———. *Medicinal Plants of the Pacific West.* Sante Fe: Red Crane Books, 1993.

Wood, Matthew. *The Book of Herbal Wisdom.* Berkeley, CA: North Atlantic Books, 1998.

SIBERIAN GINSENG

Bergner, Paul. *The Healing Power of Ginseng and the Tonic Herbs.* Rocklin, CA: Prima Publishing, 1996.

Duke, James A. *The Green Pharmacy.* Emmaus, PA: Rodale Press, 1998.

Foster, Steven. *Siberian Ginseng.* Austin, TX: American Botanical Council, 1991.

McCaleb, Rob. "Interview with I. I. Brekhman." *HerbalGram,* no. 16, spring 1988.

———. "Nature's Medicine for Memory Loss." *HerbalGram,* no. 23, summer 1990, page 15.

Weil, Andrew. *Eight Weeks to Optimum Health.* New York: Alfred A. Knopf, 1998.

Werbach, Melvyn, and Michael Murray. *Botanical Influences on Illness.* Tarzana, CA: Third Line Press, 1994. Lists multiple abstracts of clinical trials and studies.

SHIITAKE

Duke, James A. *The Green Pharmacy.* Emmaus, PA: Rodale, 1998.

Herb Research Foundation. *Herbal Immunity Boosters.* Boulder, CO: HRF, 1995.

Hobbs, Christopher. *Medicinal Mushrooms.* Capitola, CA: Botanica, 1995.

Landis, Robyn, and K. P. Khalsa. *Herbal Defense.* New York: Warner Books, 1997.

McCaleb, Rob. "Anti-Cancer Effects of Herbs." *HerbalGram,* no. 30, winter 1994, page 10.

Schmidt, M., et al. *Beyond Antibiotics.* Berkeley, CA: North Atlantic, 1994.

Werbach, Melvyn, and Michael Murray. *Botanical Influences on Illness.* Tarzana, CA: Third Line Press, 1994. Lists multiple abstracts of clinical trials and studies.

GENERAL REFERENCES

Duke, James A. *The Green Pharmacy.* Emmaus, PA: Rodale, 1998.

Ellingwood, Finley. *American Materia Medica, Therapeutics, and Pharmacognosy.* Cincinnati: Eclectic Publications, 1919.

Farnsworth, Norman. "The Present and Future of Pharmacognosy." American Botanical Council Reprint No. 209, reprinted from *American Journal of Pharmaceutical Education,* 43:239–243 (1979). World Health Organization mandate on traditional medicines.

Felter, Harvey, and John Uri Lloyd. *King's American Dispensatory.* Cincinnati: Eclectic Publications, 1895.

Herb Research Foundation. *Herbal Immunity Boosters.* Boulder,CO: HRF, 1995.

"Herbal Bacteria Busters." *Psychology and Health,* vol. 8, no. 6, November/December 1998, page 4. Essential oils of thyme, rosewood, and oregano effective in treatment of pneumonia.

Hoffmann, David. *The New Holistic Herbal.* Rockport, MA: Element, 1992.

Landis, Robyn, and K. P. Khalsa. *Herbal Defense.* New York: Warner Books, 1997.

Lifeline: "Berry Good." *USA Today,* October 8, 1998, page D1. (Cranberry juice found to prevent *E. coli* from adhering to urinary tract walls, citing *New England Journal of Medicine,* October 8, 1998.)

Medical Herbalism, all issues.

Moerman, Daniel. *Medicinal Plants of Native America.* Ann Arbor, MI: University of Michigan, Museum of Anthropology, Technical Reports, no. 19, 1986.

Moore, Michael. *Medicinal Plants of the Mountain West.* Sante Fe: Museum of New Mexico Press, 1976.

NAPRALERT Database of Botanicals Effective against Human Pathogenic Bacteria as of 12/1/1998. NAPRALERT(SM) is an acronym for Natural Products ALERT, a dynamic database that is updated periodically and which has been copyrighted from 1975 to date by the Board of Trustees, The University of Illinois. NAPRALERT(SM) is currently maintaind by the Program for Collaborative Research in the Pharmaceutical Sciences, within the Department of Medicinal Chemistry and Pharmacognosy, in the College of Pharmacy of the University of Illinois at Chicago, 833 South Wood Street (m/c 877), Chicago, IL 60612. Phone: 312-996-2246.

The data in NAPRALERT(SM) represents a synthesis of information from more than 150,000 scientific journal articles, books, abstracts, and patents, collected systematically from the global literature, since 1975.

The Protocol Journal of Botanic Medicine, all issues.

Schmidt, Michael, et al. *Beyond Antibiotics.* Berkeley, CA: North Atlantic Books, 1994.

Sparrow. "Medicine Garden Wheel." In: Buhner, Stephen (editor). *Plants of Power.* Unpublished manuscript. Use of garlic vine for malaria.

Tucker, Arthur O. "Heal Yourself With Aromatherapy." *Herbs for Health,* January/February 1999.

Weil, Andrew. *Eight Weeks to Optimum Health.* New York: Knopf, 1998.

Weiss, Rudolph. *Herbal Medicine.* Sweden: Beaconsfield, 1988.

INDEX

Bold type indicates recipe name

A

Acacia (*Acacia* spp.)
  about, 21–22
  alternatives to, 23
  preparation/dosage, 22–23
  recipes, 93, 94, 98, 105
  side effects/contraindications, 23
Aerobic bacteria, 8
Age, ginseng and, 80
Agribusiness. *See* Factory farms
AIDS, 39
Airborne Infections, Essential Oil Mix for, 99
Alcohol tinctures. *See* Tinctures, alcohol
Allicin, 33
Allium sativum. See Garlic
Aloe (*Aloe* spp.)
  about, 23–24
  alternatives to, 25
  preparation/dosage, 24
  side effects/contraindications, 24
Animal dosages, of GSE, 45
Antibacterial herbs, 63–66
Antibiotic Paradox, The (book), 4, 13
Antibiotics. *See also* Bacterial resistance;
    Botanical medicines
  development of, 3–4
  proper use of, 17
  use of, evolution of, 4–6
Antioxidants, 52–53
Appendix, 67
Artemisia absinthium. See Wormwood
Ashwagandha (*Withania somnifera*)
  about, 69–70
  alternatives to, 71
  preparation/dosage, 70
  side effects/contraindications, 70

Astragalus (*Astragalus membranaceus*)
  about, 71–72
  alternatives to, 72
  preparation/dosage, 72
  purchasing, 72
  recipes for, 73
  side effects/contraindications, 72
Astragalus Broth, 73
Athlete's foot, 96

B

Bacteremia
  causes of, 10, 11
  treatment of, 28, 63, 64
Bacterial resistance
  communication of, 8–10
  development of, 6–7
  factory farms and, 12–15
  most common drug-resistant bacteria, 11
  places of transmission, 10
  slowing emergence of, steps to, 17
  Staphylococcus aureus and, 16
Bacterial viruses, 9
Bacteriophages, defined, 9
Baginski, Bodo, 44
Bed sores, 46
Begley, Sharon, 1
Berberine, 38, 39, 40
Best Cold and Flu Tea, The, 49
Bites. *See* Venomous stings/bites
Blood infections, 10, 28, 63
Bone marrow, 67, 68
Boneset (*Eupatorium perfoliatum*)
  about, 74–76
  alternatives to, 76
  preparation/dosage, 76
  side effects/contraindications, 76

Botanical medicines. *See also* Herbal medicines; Herbs
  acacia, 21–23
  aloe, 23–25
  cryptolepsis, 25–26
  echinacea, 27–30
  eucalyptus, 30–32
  garlic, 33–36
  ginger, 36–38
  goldenseal, 38–42
  grapefruit seed extract, 42–46
  honey, 47–50
  juniper, 50–53
  licorice, 53–55
  overview, 18
  properties of, 19–20
  sage, 56–57
  usnea, 57–60
  wormwood, 60–62
Botulism, 50, 101
Branhamella catarrhalis, 101
Bread mold, 4, 5
"Breakbone fever," 74
Brigitte Mars's Herb Tea for Ear Infections, 103
Broth, Astragalus, 73
Burnet, Sir F. Macfarlane, 3
Burney, Lee, 3
Burns, treatment of, 37, 49, 50

C

Campylobacter, spread of, factory farms and, 12, 15
Capsules. *See* Powders and capsules
Ceanothus. See Red root
Chicken, 12, 14, 15
Children's ailments, preparations for
  diarrhea, 104, 105
  dosage, determining, 103
  ear infections, 100–103
  fever, 104
  glycerites and honeys, 104
Chlamydia trachomatis, 40

Citrus paradisi. See Grapefruit seed extract (GSE)
Clark's Rule, 103
Coconut Grove restaurant fire (1942), 4, 24
Cold infusions, 87
Colds and Flu, Combination Tincture Formula for, 91
Colds and Flu, Decoction for, 88
Colds and flu, treatment of, 28, 29, 30, 49
Combination Tincture Formula for Colds and Flu, 91
Coral root *(Corollorhiza maculata),* 104
Corollorhiza maculata (Coral root), 104
Cough, treatment of, 36
Cowling's Rule, 103
Cox, David, 3
Cryptolepsis *(Cryptolepsis sanguinolenta)*
  about, 25–26
  alternatives to, 26
  preparation/dosage, 26
  recipes, 94, 105
  side effects/contraindications, 26
Cryptosporidium, spread of, factory farms and, 12
Cyclospora, spread of, factory farms and, 12

D

Decoction for Colds and Flu, 88
Decoctions, making/using
  about, 87
  proportions/boiling time, 88
  recipes, 88
  red root, 78
Dengue fever, 74
Diaper rash, 96
Diarrhea
  causes of, 10, 11, 101
  treatment for, 46
  treatment of, 25, 40, 42, 65, 104, 105
Diffusers, defined, 99
Disinfectants, 46

Douches
  eucalyptus, 32
  goldenseal, 41, 42
  GSE, 46
  usnea, 59
Dried herbs, using, 90–91, 92, 104

E

Ear Infection, Oil for, 102
Ear infections
  causes of, 10, 11
  preparations for preventing, 100–101
  preparations for treating, 101–3
  treatment of, 63
Ear Infection Tincture Combination,
  102
Echinacea (*Echinacea angustifolia, E.*
  purpurea)
  about, 27–28
  alternatives to, 30
  as alternative to aloe, 25
  preparation/dosage, 29
  recipes, 91, 92, 93, 94, 96, 102
  side effects/contraindications, 29–30
Eggs, chicken, 12, 14, 15
Eight Weeks to Optimum Health (book),
  82, 83
Eleutherococcus senticosus. See Siberian
  ginseng
Emetics, 35
Enterococcus
  diseases caused by, 10, 11
  treatment of, 63
Epidemics, 4
Escherichia coli (E. coli)
  diseases caused by, 40, 41, 104
  spread of, factory farms and, 12,
    13–14, 15
  treatment of, 64
Essential Oil Mix for Airborne
  Infections, 99
Essential oils
  about, 97–100
  eucalyptus, 32

juniper, 52
  sage, 56
  wormwood, 62
Eucalyptus (*Eucalyptus* spp.)
  about, 30–31
  alternatives to, 32
  preparation/dosage, 31–32
  recipes, 89, 92, 94, 96, 98, 99, 102
  side effects/contraindications, 32
Eupatorium perfoliatum. See Boneset

F

Factory farms
  bacterial resistance and, 12–13
  E. coli, spread of, 13–14
FDA (U.S. Food and Drug
  Administration), 39
Fisher, Dr. Jeffery, 7, 12
Five-Step Herbal Regimen for an
  Ulcerated Stomach, 98
Fleming, Alexander, 3
Flu. *See* Colds and flu
Foods, for the immune system, 81–84
Formula for a Good Wound Salve, 94
Fox, Nicholas, 12, 14
Free radicals, 52–53
Fresh herbs, using, 90, 93, 104
Fungal infections, 26, 59, 96
Fungi, soil, 4, 5

G

Gargles, making/using
  eucalyptus, 32
  red root, 78
Garlic (*Allium sativum*)
  about, 33–34, 43–44, 46
  active constituents of, 19
  alternatives to, 36
  as botanical medicine, 19, 81
  odor, controlling, 34
  preparation/dosage, 35
  recipes, 93, 102
  side effects/contraindications, 35–36

Gilbert, Dr. Cynthia, 1
Ginger *(Zingiber officinale)*
    about, 36–37, 81
    alternatives to, 38
    preparation/dosage, 37
    recipes, 102
    side effects/contraindications, 38
Ginseng. *See* Siberian ginseng
Glossary, 107–9
Glycerites, 102, 104
Glycyrrhiza glabra. See Licorice
Goldenseal *(Hydrastis canadensis)*
    about, 38–41, 97
    alternatives to, 42
    as endangered plant, 41
    overuse of, 28
    preparation/dosage, 41
    recipes, 96, 98, 105
    side effects/contraindications, 42
Gonorrhea
    causes of, 10, 11
    treatment of, 63
Gram-negative bacteria, 8
Gram-positive bacteria, 8
Granulocytes, 68
Grapefruit seed extract (GSE) *(Citrus
        paradisi)*
    about, 42–44
    alternatives to, 46
    preparation/dosage, 44–46
    recipes, 92, 98, 102, 105
    side effects/contraindications, 46
GSE. *See* Grapefruit seed extract (GSE)
    (Citrus paradisi)
Gums, acacias, 21–22, 23

H

Haemophilus influenzae
    diseases caused by, 10, 11
    treatment of, 65, 101
Havel, Vaclav, 106
Healing Power of Grapefruit Seed, The
    (book), 44
Henson, Jim, 2

Herbal Materia Medica (book), 90
Herbal medicines, making/using
    alcohol tinctures, 90–92
    children's ailments, common, 100–105
    decoctions, 87–88
    essential oils, 97–100
    infusions, 85–87
    oil infusions, 92–95
    overview, 85, 86
    steams, 89
    washes, 89
    whole herbs, using, 95–97
Herbal Oil for Skin Infections, 93
Herbal Tonic Therapies (book), 55
Herbs, antibacterial
    effectiveness of, 66
    listed, 63–64
    spice blends, 65–66
    top 15, listed, 20
Herbs, for the immune system
    ashwagandha, 69–71
    astragalus, 71–73
    boneset, 74–76
    red root, 77–78
    Siberian ginseng, 79–80
Honey, wildflower
    about, 47–48
    alternatives to, 50
    as alternative to aloe, 25
    preparation/dosage, 49
    recipes, 98
    side effects/contraindications, 50
Honeys, herbal, 102, 104
Horne, Diane, 32
Hospitals, 1, 2, 10
Hot Infusion for Parasites, 87
Hot infusions, 86
Hydrastine, 38
Hydrastis canadensis. See Goldenseal

I

Immune-Enhancing Rice, 73
Immune Soup, 83

Immune system
  elements of, 67–68
  foods and vitamins for, 81–84
  herbs for strengthening, 69–80
  lifestyle choices and, 84
  revitalizing strategies, 68
Immunity, drug. See Bacterial resistance
Immunoglobulin A (IgA), 40
Impetigo, 49
Infusions, making/using
  about, 85–86
  goldenseal, 41
  oil, 92–95
  proportions/steeping time, 86
  recipes, 87
Intestinal worms, 87

J

Juniper (*Juniperus* spp.)
  about, 50–51
  alternatives to, 52–53
  preparation/dosage, 51–52
  recipes, 89, 92, 94, 96
  side effects/contraindications, 52

K

Kennedy, Donald, 9
Khalsa, K.P., 71, 73
Klebsiella pneumoniae
  diseases caused by, 10, 11
  treatment of, 64

L

Landis, Robyn, 71, 73
Lappé, Marc, 2, 4, 5, 68, 106
Lentinus edodes. See Shiitake
Levy, Dr. Stuart, 2, 4, 5, 6, 9, 13, 16, 17
Licorice (*Glycyrrhiza glabra*)
  about, 53–55
  alternatives to, 55
  preparation/dosage, 55
  recipes, 91, 98, 102, 103
  side effects/contraindications, 55

Lifestyle, immune system and, 84
Listeria, spread of, factory farms and,
  12, 15
Liver, 67, 68
Lymphocytes, 68
Lymph system, 67, 68

M

Macrophages, 68
Malaria
  causes of, 10, 11
  treatment of, 25, 26, 31, 37, 61, 65, 87
McCaleb, Rob, 71
McClintock, Barbara, 9
Meningitis, 10, 11
Methicillin-resistant *S. aureus* (MRSA), 16
Mimosas. *See* Acacia
Miracle drugs. *See* Antibiotics
Mold, bread, 4, 5
Moore, Michael, 22, 90
Mowrey, Daniel, 55
MRSA (Methicillin-resistant *S. aureus*), 16
Mushrooms, shiitake, 82, 84
Mycobacterium tuberculosis, 11, 63

N

Nasal Spray Formula for Sinus
  Infections, 92
Nasal sprays
  eucalyptus, 32
  GSE, 46
  making/using, 91–92
  usnea, 59
Neill, Marguerite, 14
Neisseria gonorrhoeae, 11, 63
Neutrophils, 68
Nonaerobic bacteria, 8

O

Oil for Ear Infection, 102
Oil infusions, making/using, 92–95
Old man's beard. *See* Usnea
Onion, as immune system booster, 81

P

Pap smear, abnormal, treatment of, 27, 29, 30
Parasites, Hot Infusion for, 87
Penicillin
  active constituents of, 19
  development of, 3, 24
Phagocytes, 68
Plague Makers, The (book), 12
Plant medicines. *See* Botanical medicines
Plasmids, 8, 10
Plasmodium falciparum, 63
Pneumonia
  causes of, 10, 11
  treatment of, 63, 64
Powders and capsules
  acacia, 23
  astragalus, 72
  cryptolepsis, 26
  echinacea, 29
  eucalyptus, 32
  garlic, 35
  ginger, 37
  goldenseal, 41
  juniper, 52
  licorice, 55
  making/using, 95, 96, 97
  red root, 78
  sage, 56
  Siberian ginseng, 80
  wormwood, 62
Pregnancy, cautions during, 42, 46, 52, 55, 62, 70, 78
Proanthocyanidin, 52, 81
Pseudomonas aeruginosa
  diseases caused by, 10, 11
  treatment of, 63

R

Red root (*Ceanothus* spp.)
  about, 77–78
  alternatives to, 78
  identifying in the wild, 78
  preparation/dosage, 78
  recipes, 91, 102
  side effects/contraindications, 78
Resistance, drug. *See* Bacterial resistance
Rice, Immune-Enhancing, 73
Rosemary Gladstar's Tea for Diarrhea, 105

S

Sage (*Salvia officinalis*)
  about, 56
  alternatives to, 57
  preparation/dosage, 56–57
  recipes, 88, 89, 92, 93
  side effects/contraindications, 57
Salmonella
  diseases caused by, 11
  spread of, factory farms and, 12, 14–15
  treatment of, 64
Salves, making/using, 94, 95
Salvia officinalis. See Sage
Scurvy, 53
Sharamon, Shalila, 44
Shigella dysenteriae
  diseases caused by, 11, 104
  spread of, factory farms and, 14, 15
  treatment of, 63
Shiitake (*Lentinus edodes*), 82, 84
Siberian ginseng (*Eleutherococcus senticosus*)
  about, 79–80
  alternatives to, 80
  compared to ashwagandha, 70
  preparation/dosage, 80
  side effects/contraindications, 80
Sinus infections, 91
Sinus Infections, Nasal Spray Formula for, 92
Skin Infections, Herbal Oil for, 93
Snuff, 41, 42
Soil fungi, 4, 5
Soup, Immune, 83
Spices, antibacterial, 65–66

Spleen, 67, 68

Spoiled: The Dangerous Truth About a Food Chain Gone Haywire (book), 12, 14

Sprays, nasal. *See* Nasal sprays

St. John's wort, 25, 50

Staphylococcus aureus
  diseases caused by, 10, 11
  drug resistance of, 3
  resistance to antibiotics, 16
  treatment of, 24, 64, 101

Steam for Upper Respiratory Infections, 89

Steams
  eucalyptus, 32
  juniper, 52
  making/using, 89

Stewart, William, 3

Strep throat, treatment of, 27, 29

Streptococcus pneumoniae
  diseases caused by, 10, 11, 27
  treatment of, 66, 101

Streptomycin, development of, 4

Suppositories, echinacea, 29

T

Teas
  acacia, 22
  astragalus, 72
  Best Cold and Flu Tea, The, 49
  boneset, 76
  Brigitte Mars's Herb Tea for Ear Infections, 103
  cryptolepsis, 26
  eucalyptus, 31
  ginger, 37
  honey, 49
  licorice, 55
  red root, 78
  Rosemary Gladstar's Tea for Diarrhea, 105
  sage, 56
  Siberian ginseng, 80
  usnea, 59
  wormwood, 62

Tea tree oil, 32

Tetracycline
  active constituents of, 19
  development of, 4, 5

Thymus, 67, 68

Tincture Combination for Diarrhea, 105

Tinctures, alcohol
  astragalus, 72
  boneset, 76
  cryptolepsis, 26
  ear infections, 102
  eucalyptus, 32
  garlic, 35
  ginger, 37
  goldenseal, 41
  licorice, 55
  making/using, 90–92
  red root, 78
  sage, 56
  Siberian ginseng, 80
  usnea, 59
  wormwood, 62

Tonsils, 67

Tuberculosis
  causes of, 10, 11
  treatment of, 63

U

Ulcers, treatment of, 48, 49, 98

United States Dept. of Agriculture (USDA), 15

United States Food and Drug Administration (FDA), 39

Upper respiratory infections, 88, 89, 91

Upper Respiratory Infections, Steam for, 89

Urinary tract infections
  causes of, 10, 11
  treatment of, 51, 63, 64

Usnea (*Usnea* spp.)
  about, 57–58
  alternatives to, 60
  preparation/dosage, 58–59
  recipes, 92, 93, 94, 96
  side effects/contraindications, 59–60